CONTENTS

INTRODUCTION

This is the age of single pot cooking where digitally controlled kitchen appliances are designed with several cooking modes to cook a variety of meals in no time. Today, finding a multipurpose cooking unit is not that of a challenge; rather, finding a perfect one for your kitchen requires a bit of a struggle, as there are unlimited options available. One brand that has earned our confidence in this regard is Ninja Foodi. Not only has the brand launched series of cooking appliances, but it keeps raising the bars by bringing new ideas to the market. The Ninja Foodi XL pro Air Fry Oven is one such innovation that has taken over the food-tech world with its amazing cooking features, a smart design, the XL size, and a multilayer cooking system.

This 10-in-1 multipurpose kitchen miracle is capable of providing a variety of cooking options all in a single device. With its efficient electric heating system, now you can bake, roast, Air fry, broil and dehydrate all types of food in no time. The user-friendly control system and its multifunctional heating mechanism make this appliance cost and time effective. If you are a foodie and love to cook a variety of meals for you and your family, then Ninja Foodi XL Pro Air Fry Oven is the right fit for you.

Before Ninja Foodi XL Air Fry Oven, cooking large portions of food in a single cooking session was really a problem for me. I had to cook in batches, which was quite time-consuming. But the Ninja Foodi XL pro Air Fry Oven has put an end to such problems; whether it's roasting full-size chicken or turkey, I can cook them easily using its WHOLE ROAST function. It can Roast, Bake, Air Fry, Toast, cook Pizza, Reheat, Broil and Dehydrate food in any of its four racks. The good news is that with the help of the recipe collection shared in this cookbook, you can create a complete menu in your Ninja Foodi XL Pro.

Ninja Foodi XL Pro Air Fry Oven

After the successful launch of its series of Air Fryer and Air Fry Ovens, Ninja Foodi has come up with its XL Pro Air Fry Oven to meet the needs of those who want to cook large servings sizes, whole turkeys, or chicken in their electric oven while trying different modes of cooking at one place. When we unbox the Ninja XL Air Fry Oven, the following are the accessories that are found along with the basic oven unit:

• Main Ninja XL Air Fry Oven

• Air fry basket

• Roast tray

• Sheet pan

• 2 wire racks

• Removable crumb tray

Air Fry Oven's Specifications:

A Ninja XL Air Fry Oven comes with the following unit specifications. All users are suggested to look into these features before bringing the unit home:

• Capacity: 12 lbs

• Dimensions in: 17.09L x 20.22W x 13.34H

• Power supply: 120V – 60Hz

• Maximum Draw: 1800 Watts

The control panel is present on the front-top portion of the oven with a glass door below it. Inside the oven, there are four layers to adjust your food. You can select "RACK LEVEL" from 1-4 after placing the food in a particular layer. Then the function key is used to select the cooking functions. The temperature and time keys are used to increase or decrease the values, and the same keys are used to set the darkness and slices of the toasts and bagels when their respective modes are selected. Once everything is set, the START and PAUSE button is used to initiate preheating and cooking.

Quick User Guide

If you are a newbie or you are setting your hands on this appliance for the first time, then here is how you can cook using its different cooking functions:

1.   First, plug in the Ninja Foodi XL pro Air Fry Oven and switch it ON. The led display will be lit up, indicating that the device is working.

2.   Since this Ninja XL pro Air Fry Oven quickly preheats, you need to prepare the food first and keep it ready for cooking before preheating.

3.   Place the Drip or crumb tray inside, at the bottom of the oven to protect its base from food particle and grease.

4.   Use the Air fryer basket, baking pan, roasting pan, or any other suitable accessory to place the food inside according to the instructions of a particular recipe.

5.   You can insert trays into any portion of this air fry oven to accommodate your food in four layers if needed and select the RACK LAYER option 1,2,3,4 from the control panel according to your need.

6.   When the food is ready, you can preheat the appliance. Close its door and select the desired cooking operation: Bake, Whole roast, Air Roast, Air Broil, Air Fry, Dehydrate, pizza, toast, bagel, or Reheat.

7.   By selecting this program, the device will show the preset temperature and cooking time on the display; you can change it by using the "+" or "- "keys for temperature and time to increase or decrease the values, respectively.

8.   If you are toasting bread or bagels, then use the temp and time keys to adjust the desired darkness of the toasts and the number of slices. The machine will automatically adjust the cooking temperature and time according to the desired darkness and set slices.

9.   Press the start button to initiate preheating. The display timer does not start ticking until the appliance is preheated. When it reaches the desired temperature, the display will show"FOOD" and beep to show if the device is preheated.

10.   Place the prepared food inside and close the lid to initiate cooking.

11.   .   Once the cooking function is completed, the device will beep to indicate that the food is now ready to serve.

APPETIZERS AND SIDE DISHES

1. Homemade Tortilla Chips

Servings: 4
Cooking Time: 55 Minutes
Ingredients:
- 1 cup flour
- Salt and black pepper to taste
- 1 tbsp golden flaxseed meal
- 2 cups shredded Cheddar cheese

Directions:
1. Melt cheddar cheese in the microwave for 1 minute. Add flour, salt, flaxseed meal, and pepper. Mix well with a fork. On a board, place the dough and knead it with hands while warm until the ingredients are well combined. Divide the dough into 2 and with a rolling pin, roll them out flat into 2 rectangles. Use a pastry cutter to cut out triangle-shaped pieces.
2. Line them in one layer on the Air Fryer basket and spray with cooking spray. Fit in the baking tray and cook for 10 minutes on Air Fry function at 400 F. Serve with a cheese dip.

2. Drunken Peas

Servings: 4
Cooking Time: 7 Minutes
Ingredients:
- 1 pound fresh peas
- 4 ounces smoked pancetta, chopped
- 1 green onion, sliced
- ¼ cup beer
- 1 tablespoon fresh mint, chopped
- 1 tablespoon butter
- Salt and ground black pepper, to taste
- 2 cups water

Directions:
1. Place the water in the instant jug, place the steam basket and set aside. In a heat-resistant skillet, mix the bacon with half the onion and spread over the bottom.
2. Heat on the stove over medium-high heat for 3 minutes, add beer, peas and salt, stir and remove from heat. Cover this pan with aluminum foil, place it in the steam basket, cover the Instant Pot and cook for 1 minute in the Manual setting.
3. Relieve the pressure, uncover the pan, add salt, pepper, mint and butter, mix, divide between the dishes and serve with the rest of the onion sprinkled on top.
- **Nutrition Info:** Calories: 134, Fat: 2, Fiber: 2.5, Carbohydrate: 10, Proteins: 4.3

3. Air Fried Mac & Cheese

Servings: 1
Cooking Time: 15 Minutes
Ingredients:
- 1 cup cooked macaroni
- 1 cup grated cheddar cheese
- ½ cup warm milk
- 1 tbsp Parmesan cheese
- Salt and black pepper to taste

Directions:
1. Preheat on Air Fry function to 350 F. Add the macaroni to Air Fryer baking pan. Stir in the cheddar cheese and milk. Season with salt and pepper. Place the dish in the toaster oven and cook for 10 minutes. Sprinkle with Parmesan cheese and serve.

4. Air Fryer Chicken Breasts

Servings:4
Cooking Time: 30 Minutes
Ingredients:
- 4 chicken breasts
- 1 tbsp olive oil
- Salt and black pepper to taste
- 1 tsp garlic powder

Directions:
1. Brush the breasts with olive oil and season with salt, garlic powder, and black pepper. Arrange the breasts on the frying basket. Select AirFry function, adjust the temperature to 380 F, and press Start. Cook for 20 minutes until nice and crispy. Serve warm.

5. Chickpeas With Rosemary & Sage

Servings: 4
Cooking Time: 20 Minutes
Ingredients:
- 2 (14.5-ounce) cans chickpeas, rinsed
- 2 tbsp olive oil
- 1 tsp dried rosemary
- ½ tsp dried thyme
- ¼ tsp dried sage
- ¼ tsp salt

Directions:
1. In a bowl, mix together chickpeas, oil, rosemary, thyme, sage, and salt. Transfer them to the Air Fryer baking dish and spread in an even layer. Cook for 15 minutes at 380 F on Bake function, shaking once halfway through cooking. Serve.

6. Wonton Poppers

Servings: 10
Cooking Time: 10 Minutes
Ingredients:
- Nonstick cooking spray
- 1 package refrigerated square wonton wrappers
- 1 8-ounce package cream cheese, softened

- 3 jalapenos, seeds and ribs removed, finely chopped
- 1/2 cup shredded cheddar cheese

Directions:
1. Place baking pan in position 2 of the oven. Lightly spray fryer basket with cooking spray.
2. In a large bowl, combine all ingredients except the wrappers until combined.
3. Lay wrappers in a single layer on a baking sheet. Spoon a teaspoon of filling in the center. Moisten the edges with water and fold wrappers over filling, pinching edges to seal. Place in a single layer in the basket.
4. Place the basket in the oven and set to air fry on 375°F for 10 minutes. Cook until golden brown and crisp, turning over halfway through cooking time. Repeat with remaining ingredients. Serve immediately.

- **Nutrition Info:** Calories 287, Total Fat 11g, Saturated Fat 6g, Total Carbs 38g, Net Carbs 37g, Protein 9g, Sugar 1g, Fiber 1g, Sodium 485mg, Potassium 98mg, Phosphorus 104mg

7. Buttered Corn

Servings: 2
Cooking Time: 20 Minutes
Ingredients:
- 2 corn on the cob
- Salt and freshly ground black pepper, as needed
- 2 tablespoons butter, softened and divided

Directions:
1. Sprinkle the cobs evenly with salt and black pepper.
2. Then, rub with 1 tablespoon of butter.
3. With 1 piece of foil, wrap each cob.
4. Press "Power Button" of Air Fry Oven and turn the dial to select the "Air Fry" mode.
5. Press the Time button and again turn the dial to set the cooking time to 20 minutes.
6. Now push the Temp button and rotate the dial to set the temperature at 320 degrees F.
7. Press "Start/Pause" button to start.
8. When the unit beeps to show that it is preheated, open the lid.
9. Arrange the cobs in "Air Fry Basket" and insert in the oven.
10. Serve warm.

- **Nutrition Info:** Calories 186 Total Fat 12.2 g Saturated Fat 7.4 g Cholesterol 31 mg Sodium 163 mg Total Carbs 20.1 g Fiber 2.5 g Sugar 3.2g Protein 2.9 g

8. Yogurt Masala Cashew

Servings: 2
Cooking Time: 25 Minutes
Ingredients:
- 8 oz Greek yogurt

- 2 tbsp mango powder
- 8¾ oz cashew nuts
- Salt and black pepper to taste
- 1 tsp coriander powder
- ½ tsp masala powder
- ½ tsp black pepper powder

Directions:
1. Preheat on Air Fry function to 350 F. In a bowl, mix all powders, salt, and pepper. Add in cashews and toss to coat thoroughly. Place the cashews in your Air Fryer baking pan and cook for 15 minutes, shaking every 5 minutes. Serve.

9. Baked Potatoes With Yogurt And Chives

Servings:4
Cooking Time: 35 Minutes
Ingredients:
- 4 (7-ounce / 198-g) russet potatoes, rinsed
- Olive oil spray
- ½ teaspoon kosher salt, divided
- ½ cup 2% plain Greek yogurt
- ¼ cup minced fresh chives
- Freshly ground black pepper, to taste

Directions:
1. Pat the potatoes dry and pierce them all over with a fork. Spritz the potatoes with olive oil spray. Sprinkle with ¼ teaspoon of the salt.
2. Transfer the potatoes to the baking pan.
3. Slide the baking pan into Rack Position 1, select Convection Bake, set temperature to 400ºF (205ºC), and set time to 35 minutes.
4. When cooking is complete, the potatoes should be fork-tender. Remove from the oven and split open the potatoes. Top with the yogurt, chives, the remaining ¼ teaspoon of salt, and finish with the black pepper. Serve immediately.

10. Garlic & Parmesan Bread Bites

Servings: 12
Cooking Time: 7 Minutes
Ingredients:
- 2 ciabatta loaves
- 1 stick butter at room temperature
- 4-6 crushed garlic cloves
- Chopped parsley
- 2 tablespoons finely grated parmesan

Directions:
1. Start by cutting bread in half and toasting it crust-side down for 2 minutes.
2. Mix the butter, garlic, and parsley together and spread over the bread.
3. Sprinkle parmesan over bread and toast in oven another 5 minutes.

- **Nutrition Info:** Calories: 191, Sodium: 382 mg, Dietary Fiber: 1.0 g, Total Fat: 9.4 g, Total Carbs: 21.7 g, Protein: 4.9 g.

11. Cheese & Zucchini Cake With Yogurt

Servings:4
Cooking Time: 20 Minutes
Ingredients:
- 1 ½ cups flour
- 1 tsp cinnamon
- 3 eggs
- 1 tsp baking powder
- 2 tbsp sugar
- 1 cup milk
- 2 tbsp butter, melted
- 1 tbsp yogurt
- ½ cup zucchini, shredded
- A pinch of salt
- 2 tbsp cream cheese, softened

Directions:
1. In a bowl, whisk eggs with sugar, salt, cinnamon, cream cheese, flour, and baking powder. In another bowl, combine all of the liquid ingredients. Gently combine the dry and liquid mixtures.
2. Stir in zucchini. Line the muffin tins with baking paper and pour in the batter. Arrange on a baking tray and place in the oven. Press Start and cook for 15 minutes. Serve chilled.

12. Cheesy Broccoli Bites

Servings: 5
Cooking Time: 12 Minutes
Ingredients:
- 1 cup broccoli florets
- 1 egg, beaten
- ¾ cup cheddar cheese, grated
- 2 tablespoons Parmesan cheese, grated
- ¾ cup panko breadcrumbs
- Salt and freshly ground black pepper, as needed

Directions:
1. In a food processor, add the broccoli and pulse until finely crumbled.
2. In a large bowl, mix together the broccoli, and remaining ingredients.
3. Make small equal-sized balls from the mixture.
4. Press "Power Button" of Air Fry Oven and turn the dial to select the "Air Fry" mode.
5. Press the Time button and again turn the dial to set the cooking time to 12 minutes.
6. Now push the Temp button and rotate the dial to set the temperature at 350 degrees F.
7. Press "Start/Pause" button to start.
8. When the unit beeps to show that it is preheated, open the lid.

9. Arrange the broccoli balls in "Air Fry Basket" and insert in the oven.
10. Serve warm.
- **Nutrition Info:** Calories 153 Total Fat 8.2 g Saturated Fat 4.5g Cholesterol 52 mg Sodium 172 mg Total Carbs 4 g Fiber 0.5 g Sugar 0.5 g Protein 7.1 g

13. Charred Green Beans With Sesame Seeds

Servings:4
Cooking Time: 8 Minutes
Ingredients:
- 1 tablespoon reduced-sodium soy sauce or tamari
- ½ tablespoon Sriracha sauce
- 4 teaspoons toasted sesame oil, divided
- 12 ounces (340 g) trimmed green beans
- ½ tablespoon toasted sesame seeds

Directions:
1. Whisk together the soy sauce, Sriracha sauce, and 1 teaspoon of sesame oil in a small bowl until smooth. Set aside.
2. Toss the green beans with the remaining sesame oil in a large bowl until evenly coated.
3. Place the green beans in the air fryer basket in a single layer.
4. Put the air fryer basket on the baking pan and slide into Rack Position 2, select Air Fry, set temperature to 375ºF (190ºC), and set time to 8 minutes.
5. Stir the green beans halfway through the cooking time.
6. When cooking is complete, the green beans should be lightly charred and tender. Remove from the oven to a platter. Pour the prepared sauce over the top of green beans and toss well. Serve sprinkled with the toasted sesame seeds.

14. Crispy Zucchini Sticks

Servings:4
Cooking Time: 14 Minutes
Ingredients:
- 2 small zucchini, cut into 2-inch × ½-inch sticks
- 3 tablespoons chickpea flour
- 2 teaspoons arrowroot (or cornstarch)
- ½ teaspoon garlic granules
- ¼ teaspoon sea salt
- ⅛ teaspoon freshly ground black pepper
- 1 tablespoon water
- Cooking spray

Directions:
1. Combine the zucchini sticks with the chickpea flour, arrowroot, garlic granules, salt, and pepper in a medium bowl and toss to coat. Add the water and stir to mix well.

2. Spritz the air fryer basket with cooking spray and spread out the zucchini sticks in the pan. Mist the zucchini sticks with cooking spray.
3. Put the air fryer basket on the baking pan and slide into Rack Position 2, select Air Fry, set temperature to 392ºF (200ºC), and set time to 14 minutes.
4. Stir the sticks halfway through the cooking time.
5. When cooking is complete, the zucchini sticks should be crispy and nicely browned. Remove from the oven and serve warm.

15. Spinach And Goat Cheese Risotto

Servings: 6
Cooking Time: 10 Minutes
Ingredients:
- ¾ cup yellow onion, chopped
- 1½ cups Arborio rice
- 12 ounces spinach, chopped
- 3½ cups hot vegetable stock
- ½ cup white wine
- 2 garlic cloves, peeled and minced
- 2 tablespoons extra virgin olive oil
- Salt and ground black pepper, to taste
- ⅓ cup pecans, toasted and chopped
- 4 ounces goat cheese, soft and crumbled
- 2 tablespoons lemon juice

Directions:
1. Put the Instant Pot in the sauté mode, add the oil and heat. Add garlic and onion, mix and cook for 5 minutes.
2. Add the rice, mix and cook for 1 minute. Add wine, stir and cook until it is absorbed. Add 3 cups of stock, cover the Instant Pot and cook the rice for 4 minutes.
3. Release the pressure, uncover the Instant Pot, add the spinach, stir and cook for 3 minutes in Manual mode. Add salt, pepper, the rest of the stock, lemon juice and goat cheese and mix. Divide between plates, decorate with nuts and serve.
- **Nutrition Info:** Calories: 340, Fat: 23, Fiber: 4.5, Carbohydrate: 24, Proteins: 18.9

16. Paprika Potatoes

Servings: 4
Cooking Time: 30 Minutes
Ingredients:
- 1 lb baby potatoes, quartered
- 1/4 tsp rosemary, crushed
- 1/2 tsp thyme
- 2 tbsp paprika
- 2 tbsp coconut oil, melted
- 1 tbsp olive oil
- Pepper
- Salt

Directions:

1. Fit the oven with the rack in position
2. Place potatoes in a baking dish and sprinkle with paprika, rosemary, thyme, pepper, and salt.
3. Drizzle with oil and melted coconut oil.
4. Set to bake at 425 F for 35 minutes. After 5 minutes place the baking dish in the preheated oven.
5. Serve and enjoy.
- **Nutrition Info:** Calories 165 Fat 10.9 g Carbohydrates 16.2 g Sugar 0.4 g Protein 3.4 g Cholesterol 0 mg

17. French Fries

Servings: 4
Cooking Time: 10 Minutes
Ingredients:
- ¼ teaspoon baking soda Oil for frying
- Salt, to taste
- 8 medium potatoes, peeled, cut into medium matchsticks, and patted dry
- 1 cup water

Directions:
1. Put the water in the Instant Pot, add the salt and baking soda and mix. Place the potatoes in the steam basket and place them in the Instant Pot, cover and cook with manual adjustment for 3 minutes.
2. Release the pressure naturally, remove the chips from the Instant Pot and place them in a bowl. Heat a pan with enough oil over medium-high heat, add the potatoes, spread and cook until they are golden brown.
3. Transfer the potatoes to the paper towels to drain the excess fat and place them in a bowl. Salt, mix well and serve.
- **Nutrition Info:** Calories: 300, Fat: 10, Fiber: 3.7, Carbohydrate: 41, Proteins: 3.4

18. Roasted Garlic(3)

Servings: 12 Cloves
Cooking Time: 20 Minutes
Ingredients:
- 1 medium head garlic
- 2 tsp. avocado oil

Directions:
1. Remove any hanging excess peel from the garlic but leave the cloves covered. Cut off ¼ of the head of garlic, exposing the tips of the cloves
2. Drizzle with avocado oil. Place the garlic head into a small sheet of aluminum foil, completely enclosing it. Place it into the air fryer basket. Adjust the temperature to 400 Degrees F and set the timer for 20 minutes. If your garlic head is a bit smaller, check it after 15 minutes
3. When done, garlic should be golden brown and very soft

4. To serve, cloves should pop out and easily be spread or sliced. Store in an airtight container in the refrigerator up to 5 days.
5. You may also freeze individual cloves on a baking sheet, then store together in a freezer-safe storage bag once frozen.
- **Nutrition Info:** Calories: 11; Protein: 2g; Fiber: 1g; Fat: 7g; Carbs: 0g

19. Tasty Butternut Squash

Servings: 4
Cooking Time: 15 Minutes
Ingredients:
- 4 cups butternut squash, cut into 1-inch pieces
- 1 tbsp brown sugar
- 2 tbsp olive oil
- 1 tsp Chinese 5 spice powder

Directions:
1. Fit the oven with the rack in position 2.
2. Toss squash into the bowl with remaining ingredients.
3. Transfer squash in the air fryer basket then places the air fryer basket in the baking pan.
4. Place a baking pan on the oven rack. Set to air fry at 400 F for 15 minutes.
5. Serve and enjoy.
- **Nutrition Info:** Calories 132 Fat 7.1 g Carbohydrates 18.6 g Sugar 5.3 g Protein 1.4 g Cholesterol 0 mg

20. Crispy Onion Rings With Buttermilk

Servings: 4
Cooking Time: 30 Minutes
Ingredients:
- 2 sweet onions
- 2 cups buttermilk
- 2 cups pancake mix
- 2 cups water
- 1 package cornbread mix
- 1 tsp salt

Directions:
1. Preheat on Air Fry function to 370 F. Slice the onions into rings. Combine the pancake mix with water. Line a baking sheet with parchment paper. Dip the rings in the cornbread mixture first, and then in the pancake batter.
2. Place the onion rings onto the greased basket and then into the baking tray. Cook for 8-12 minutes, flipping once until crispy. Serve with salsa rosa.

21. Roasted Curried Cauliflower

Servings: 4
Cooking Time: 35 Minutes
Ingredients:
- 1-1/2 tablespoons extra-virgin olive oil
- 1 teaspoon mustard seeds
- 1 teaspoon cumin seeds
- 3/4 teaspoon curry powder
- 3/4 teaspoon coarse salt
- 1 large head cauliflower
- Olive oil cooking spray

Directions:
1. Start by preheating toaster oven to 375°F.
2. Combine curry, mustard, cumin, and salt in a large bowl.
3. Break cauliflower into pieces and add it to the bowl.
4. Toss contents of bowl until the cauliflower is completely covered in the spice mix.
5. Coat a baking sheet in olive oil spray and lay cauliflower in a single layer over the sheet.
6. Roast for 35 minutes.
- **Nutrition Info:** Calories: 105, Sodium: 64 mg, Dietary Fiber: 5.6 g, Total Fat: 5.9 g, Total Carbs: 11.9 g, Protein: 4.5 g.

22. Easy Broccoli Bread

Servings: 6
Cooking Time: 30 Minutes
Ingredients:
- 5 eggs, lightly beaten
- 3/4 cup broccoli florets, chopped
- 2 tsp baking powder
- 3 1/1 tbsp coconut flour
- 1 cup cheddar cheese, shredded

Directions:
1. Fit the oven with the rack in position
2. Add all ingredients into the bowl and mix well.
3. Pour egg mixture into the greased loaf pan.
4. Set to bake at 350 F for 35 minutes. After 5 minutes place the loaf pan in the preheated oven.
5. Cut the loaf into the slices and serve.
- **Nutrition Info:** Calories 174 Fat 11.3 g Carbohydrates 7.4 g Sugar 1.2 g Protein 11 g Cholesterol 156 mg

23. Garlicky Potatoes

Servings: 4
Cooking Time: 6 Minutes
Ingredients:
- Salt and ground black pepper, to taste
- 1 pound new potatoes, peeled and sliced thin
- 1 cup water
- 1 tablespoon extra-virgin olive oil
- 2 garlic cloves, peeled and minced
- ¼ teaspoon dried rosemary

Directions:
1. Place the potatoes and water in the Instant Pot steamer basket, cover and cook for 4 minutes in manual mode. In a heat-resistant dish, mix the rosemary with olive oil and garlic, cover and microwave for 1 minute.

2. Release the pressure from the Instant Pot, drain the potatoes and spread them over an upholstered pan. Add the oil, salt and pepper mixture, mix to cover, divide between the plates and serve.
- **Nutrition Info:** Calories: 94, Fat: 1, Fiber: 2.2, Carbohydrate: 21, Proteins: 2.5

24. Healthy Parsnip Fries

Servings:3
Cooking Time: 20 Minutes
Ingredients:
- 4 large parsnips, sliced
- ¼ cup flour
- ¼ cup olive oil
- ¼ cup water
- A pinch of salt

Directions:
1. Preheat on AirFry function to 390 F. In a bowl, mix the flour, olive oil, water, and parsnip slices. Mix well and toss to coat.
2. Arrange the fries on the frying basket and place in the oven. Press Start and cook for 15 minutes. Serve with yogurt and garlic paste.

25. Tasty Saffron Risotto

Servings: 10
Cooking Time: 10 Minutes
Ingredients:
- 2 tablespoons extra virgin olive oil
- ½ cup onion, peeled and chopped
- 2 tablespoons hot milk
- ½ teaspoon saffron threads, crushed
- 1½ cups Arborio rice
- 3½ cups vegetable stock
- Salt, to taste
- 1 cinnamon stick
- ⅓ cup dried currants
- 1 tablespoon honey
- ⅓ cup almonds, chopped

Directions:
1. In a bowl, mix the milk with the saffron, mix and set aside. Put the Instant Pot in the sauté mode, add the oil and heat.
2. Add the onion, mix and cook for 5 minutes. Add rice, broth, saffron and milk, honey, salt, almonds, cinnamon stick and blackcurrant. Stir, cover the Instant Pot and cook over rice for 5 minutes.
3. Relieve the pressure, add rice to the rice, discard the cinnamon stick, divide it between the plates and serve.
- **Nutrition Info:** Calories: 260, Fat: 7, Fiber: 2, Carbohydrate: 41, Sugar: 1.5, Proteins: 3.9

26. Cabbage Wedges With Parmesan

Servings: 4

Cooking Time: 30 Minutes
Ingredients:
- ½ head of cabbage, cut into 4 wedges
- 4 tbsp butter, melted
- 2 cups Parmesan cheese, grated
- Salt and black pepper to taste
- 1 tsp smoked paprika

Directions:
1. Preheat on Air Fry function to 330 F. Line a baking sheet with parchment paper. Brush the cabbage wedges with the butter. Season with salt and pepper.
2. Coat cabbage with Parmesan cheese and arrange on the baking pan; sprinkle with paprika. Cook for 15 minutes, flip, and cook for an additional 10 minutes. Serve with yogurt dip.

27. Green Beans And Mushrooms

Servings: 4
Cooking Time: 6 Minutes
Ingredients:
- 1 small yellow onion, peeled and chopped
- 6 ounces bacon, chopped
- Salt and ground black pepper, to taste Balsamic vinegar
- 1-pound fresh green beans, trimmed
- 1 garlic clove, peeled and minced
- 8 ounces mushrooms, sliced

Directions:
1. Place the beans in the Instant Pot, add water to cover them, cover the Instant Pot and cook for 3 minutes in manual configuration.
2. Release the pressure naturally, drain the beans and set aside. Place the Instant Pot in the sauté mode, add the bacon and sauté for 1 to 2 minutes, stirring constantly.
3. Add garlic and onion, mix and cook 2 minutes. Add the mushrooms, mix and cook until tender. Add the drain beans, salt, pepper and a pinch of vinegar, mix, remove from heat, divide between plates and serve.
- **Nutrition Info:** Calories: 120, Fat: 3.7, Fiber: 3.3, Carbohydrate: 7.5, Proteins: 2.4

28. Crunchy Parmesan Snack Mix

Servings: 6 Cups
Cooking Time: 6 Minutes
Ingredients:
- 2 cups oyster crackers
- 2 cups Chex rice
- 1 cup sesame sticks
- ⅔ cup finely grated Parmesan cheese
- 8 tablespoons unsalted butter, melted
- 1½ teaspoons granulated garlic
- ½ teaspoon kosher salt

Directions:

1. Toss together all the ingredients in a large bowl until well coated. Spread the mixture in the baking pan in an even layer.
2. Slide the baking pan into Rack Position 1, select Convection Bake, set temperature to 350ºF (180ºC) and set time to 6 minutes.
3. After 3 minutes, remove from the oven and stir the mixture. Return to the oven and continue cooking.
4. When cooking is complete, the mixture should be lightly browned and fragrant. Let cool before serving.

29. Garlic Lemon Roasted Chicken

Servings: 4
Cooking Time: 60 Minutes
Ingredients:
- 1 (3 ½ pounds) whole chicken
- 2 tbsp olive oil
- Salt and black pepper to taste
- 1 lemon, cut into quarters
- 5 garlic cloves

Directions:
1. Preheat on Air Fry function to 360 F. Brush the chicken with olive oil and season with salt and pepper. Stuff with lemon and garlic cloves into the cavity.
2. Place the chicken breast-side down onto the Air Fryer basket. Tuck the legs and wings tips under. Fit in the baking tray and cook for 45 minutes at 350 F on Bake function. Let rest for 5-6 minutes, then carve and serve.

30. Cheesy Squash Casserole

Servings: 6
Cooking Time: 30 Minutes
Ingredients:
- 2 lbs yellow summer squash, cut into chunks
- 1/2 cup liquid egg substitute
- 3/4 cup cheddar cheese, shredded
- 1/4 cup mayonnaise
- 1/4 tsp salt

Directions:
1. Fit the oven with the rack in position
2. Add squash in a saucepan then pour enough water in a saucepan to cover the squash. Bring to boil.
3. Turn heat to medium and cook for 10 minutes or until tender. Drain well.
4. In a large mixing bowl, combine together squash, egg substitute, mayonnaise, 1/2 cup cheese, and salt.
5. Transfer squash mixture into a greased baking dish.
6. Set to bake at 375 F for 35 minutes. After 5 minutes place the baking dish in the preheated oven.
7. Sprinkle remaining cheese on top.

8. Serve and enjoy.
- **Nutrition Info:** Calories 130 Fat 8.2 g Carbohydrates 7.7 g Sugar 3.5 g Protein 8 g Cholesterol 18 mg

31. Mustard Chicken Wings

Servings:4
Cooking Time: 30 Minutes
Ingredients:
- ½ tsp celery salt
- ½ tsp bay leaf powder
- ½ tsp ground black pepper
- ½ tsp paprika
- ¼ tsp dry mustard
- ¼ tsp cayenne pepper
- ¼ tsp allspice
- 2 pounds chicken wings

Directions:
1. Preheat to 400 F on AirFry function. In a bowl, mix celery salt, bay leaf powder, black pepper, paprika, dry mustard, cayenne pepper, and allspice. Add in the wings and toss to coat.
2. Arrange the wings in an even layer on the basket. Press Start and AirFry the chicken until it's no longer pink around the bone, about 20-25 minutes until crispy on the outside. Serve.

32. Cheese Biscuits

Servings:6
Cooking Time: 35 Minutes
Ingredients:
- ½ cup + 1 tbsp butter
- 2 tbsp sugar
- 3 cups flour
- 1 ⅓ cups buttermilk
- ½ cup cheddar cheese, grated

Directions:
1. Preheat on AirFry function to 380 F. Lay a parchment paper on a baking plate. In a bowl, mix sugar, flour, ½ cup butter, cheese, and buttermilk to form a batter. Make balls from the batter and roll in the flour. Place the balls in the baking plate and flatten into biscuit shapes. Sprinkle with cheese and the remaining butter. Place in the oven and press Start. Cook for 30 minutes, tossing every 10 minutes. Serve chilled.

33. Honey Corn Muffins

Servings: 8
Cooking Time: 20 Minutes
Ingredients:
- 2 eggs
- 1/2 cup sugar
- 1 1/4 cups self-rising flour
- 3/4 cup yellow cornmeal
- 1/2 cup butter, melted

- 3/4 cup buttermilk
- 1 tbsp honey

Directions:
1. Fit the oven with the rack in position
2. Spray 8-cups muffin tin with cooking spray and set aside.
3. In a large bowl, mix together cornmeal, sugar, and flour.
4. In a separate bowl, whisk the eggs with buttermilk and honey until well combined.
5. Slowly add egg mixture and melted butter to the cornmeal mixture and stir until just mixed.
6. Spoon batter into the prepared muffin tin.
7. Set to bake at 350 F for 25 minutes. After 5 minutes place muffin tin in the preheated oven.
8. Serve and enjoy.
- **Nutrition Info:** Calories 294 Fat 13.4 g Carbohydrates 39.6 g Sugar 16 g Protein 5.2 g Cholesterol 72 mg

34. Parmesan Baked Asparagus

Servings: 4
Cooking Time: 12 Minutes
Ingredients:
- 1 lb asparagus, wash, trimmed, and cut the ends
- 1 tbsp dried parsley
- 2 garlic cloves, minced
- 2 tbsp olive oil
- 3 oz parmesan cheese, shaved
- 1 tsp dried oregano
- Pepper
- Salt

Directions:
1. Fit the oven with the rack in position
2. Arrange asparagus in baking pan. Drizzle with olive oil and season with pepper and salt.
3. Spread cheese, oregano, parsley, and garlic over the asparagus
4. Set to bake at 425 F for 17 minutes. After 5 minutes place the baking pan in the preheated oven.
5. Serve and enjoy.
- **Nutrition Info:** Calories 155 Fat 11.8 g Carbohydrates 6 g Sugar 2.2 g Protein 9.5 g Cholesterol 15 mg

35. Crunchy Cheese Twists

Servings: 8
Cooking Time: 45 Minutes
Ingredients:
- 2 cups cauliflower florets, steamed
- 1 egg
- 3 ½ oz oats
- 1 red onion, diced
- 1 tsp mustard

- 5 oz cheddar cheese, shredded
- Salt and black pepper to taste

Directions:
1. Preheat on Air Fry function to 350 F. Place the oats in a food processor and pulse until they are the consistency of breadcrumbs.
2. Place the cauliflower florets in a large bowl. Add in the rest of the ingredients and mix to combine. Take a little bit of the mixture and twist it into a straw.
3. Place onto a lined baking tray and repeat the process with the rest of the mixture. Cook for 10 minutes, turn over, and cook for an additional 10 minutes. Serve.

36. Gourmet Beef Sticks

Servings: 3
Cooking Time: 10 Minutes + Chilling Time
Ingredients:
- 1 lb ground beef
- 3 tbsp sugar
- A pinch garlic powder
- A pinch chili powder
- Salt to taste
- 1 tsp liquid smoke

Directions:
1. Place the beef, sugar, garlic powder, chili powder, salt and liquid smoke in a bowl. Mix well. Mold out 4 sticks with your hands, place them on a plate, and refrigerate for 30 minutes.
2. Remove and cook in the oven at 350 F for 10 minutes on Bake function. Flip and continue cooking for another 5 minutes until browned.

37. Mom's Tarragon Chicken Breast Packets

Servings: 2
Cooking Time: 15 Minutes
Ingredients:
- 2 chicken breasts
- 1 tbsp butter
- Salt and black pepper to taste
- ¼ tsp dried tarragon

Directions:
1. Preheat on Bake function to 380 F. Place each chicken breast on a 12x12 inches foil wrap. Top the chicken with tarragon and butter; season with salt and pepper. Wrap the foil around the chicken breast in a loose way to create a flow of air. Cook the in your oven for 15 minutes. Carefully unwrap and serve.

38. Butternut Squash Croquettes

Servings:4
Cooking Time: 17 Minutes
Ingredients:

- $^1/_3$ butternut squash, peeled and grated
- $^1/_3$ cup all-purpose flour
- 2 eggs, whisked
- 4 cloves garlic, minced
- 1½ tablespoons olive oil
- 1 teaspoon fine sea salt
- $^1/_3$ teaspoon freshly ground black pepper, or more to taste
- $^1/_3$ teaspoon dried sage
- A pinch of ground allspice

Directions:
1. Line the air fryer basket with parchment paper. Set aside.
2. In a mixing bowl, stir together all the ingredients until well combined.
3. Make the squash croquettes: Use a small cookie scoop to drop tablespoonfuls of the squash mixture onto a lightly floured surface and shape into balls with your hands. Transfer them to the basket.
4. Put the air fryer basket on the baking pan and slide into Rack Position 2, select Air Fry, set temperature to 345ºF (174ºC), and set time to 17 minutes.
5. When cooking is complete, the squash croquettes should be golden brown. Remove from the oven to a plate and serve warm.

39. Brussels Sprouts & Sweet Potatoes

Servings: 6
Cooking Time: 15 Minutes
Ingredients:
- 1 lb sweet potatoes, peeled and diced into 1/2-inch cubes
- 1 lb Brussels sprouts, remove stem & into quartered
- 2 tbsp olive oil
- 1 tsp chili powder
- Pepper
- Salt

Directions:
1. Fit the oven with the rack in position 2.
2. Add Brussels sprouts, sweet potatoes, chili powder, olive oil, pepper, and salt into the mixing bowl and toss well.
3. Transfer Brussels sprouts & sweet potato mixture in air fryer basket then place air fryer basket in baking pan.
4. Place a baking pan on the oven rack. Set to air fry at 380 F for 15 minutes.
5. Serve and enjoy.
- **Nutrition Info:** Calories 163 Fat 5.1 g Carbohydrates 28.2 g Sugar 2 g Protein 3.8 g Cholesterol 0 mg

40. Mixed Nuts With Cinnamon

Servings: 4
Cooking Time: 25 Minutes

Ingredients:
- ½ cup pecans
- ½ cup walnuts
- ½ cup almonds
- A pinch cayenne pepper
- 2 tbsp sugar
- 2 tbsp egg whites
- 2 tsp cinnamon

Directions:
1. Add the pepper, sugar, and cinnamon to a bowl and mix well; set aside. In another bowl, combine the pecans, walnuts, almonds, and egg whites. Add the spice mixture to the nuts and give it a good mix. Lightly grease the baking tray with cooking spray.
2. Pour in the nuts and cook for 10 minutes on Bake function at 350 F. Shake and cook for further for 10 minutes. Pour the nuts in a bowl. Let cool before serving.

41. Healthy Asparagus Potatoes

Servings: 4
Cooking Time: 35 Minutes
Ingredients:
- 9 oz asparagus, cut into 2-inch pieces
- 2 lbs potatoes, cut into quarters
- 1/4 cup balsamic vinegar
- 2 tbsp olive oil

Directions:
1. Fit the oven with the rack in position
2. In a large bowl, add potatoes, balsamic vinegar, olive oil, and salt and toss well.
3. Spread potatoes in baking pan.
4. Set to bake at 390 F for 25 minutes. After 5 minutes place the baking pan in the preheated oven.
5. Add asparagus and stir well and bake for 15 minutes more.
6. Season with pepper and salt.
7. Serve and enjoy.
- **Nutrition Info:** Calories 232 Fat 7.3 g Carbohydrates 38.3 g Sugar 3.9 g Protein 5.2 g Cholesterol 0 mg

42. French Beans With Toasted Almonds

Servings: 4
Cooking Time: 25 Minutes
Ingredients:
- 1 ½ lb French beans, trimmed
- Salt and black pepper to taste
- ½ pound shallots, chopped
- 3 tbsp olive oil
- ½ cup almonds, toasted

Directions:
1. Preheat on Air Fry function to 400 F. Blanch the French beans in filled with water pot over medium heat until tender, about 5-6 minutes. Remove with slotted spoon toa

bowl and mix in olive oil, shallots, salt, and pepper. Add the mixture to a baking dish and cook in your for 10 minutes, shaking once or twice. Serve sprinkled with almonds.

43. Maple Shrimp With Coconut

Servings: 3
Cooking Time: 30 Minutes
Ingredients:
- 1 lb jumbo shrimp, peeled and deveined
- ¾ cup shredded coconut
- 1 tbsp maple syrup
- ½ cup breadcrumbs
- ⅓ cup cornstarch
- ½ cup milk

Directions:
1. Pour the cornstarch in a zipper bag, add shrimp, zip the bag up and shake vigorously to coat with the cornstarch. Mix the syrup and milk in a bowl and set aside.
2. In a separate bowl, mix the breadcrumbs and shredded coconut. Open the zipper bag and remove each shrimp while shaking off excess starch. Dip shrimp in the milk mixture and then in the crumb mixture while pressing loosely to trap enough crumbs and coconut.
3. Place in the basket without overcrowding and fit in the baking tray. Cook for 12 minutes at 350 F on Air Fry function, flipping once halfway through until golden brown. Serve warm.

44. Baked Eggplant Pepper & Mushrooms

Servings: 4
Cooking Time: 20 Minutes
Ingredients:
- 2 eggplants
- 2 cups mushrooms
- 1/4 tsp black pepper
- 4 bell peppers
- 2 tbsp olive oil
- 1 tsp salt

Directions:
1. Fit the oven with the rack in position
2. Cut all vegetables into the small bite-sized pieces and place in a baking dish.
3. Drizzle vegetables with olive oil and season with pepper and salt.
4. Set to bake at 390 F for 25 minutes. After 5 minutes place the baking dish in the preheated oven.
5. Serve and enjoy.
- **Nutrition Info:** Calories 87 Fat 4 g Carbohydrates 13.2 g Sugar 7.4 g Protein 2.5 g Cholesterol 0 mg

45. Allspice Chicken Wings

Servings: 4
Cooking Time: 45 Minutes
Ingredients:
- ½ tsp celery salt
- ½ tsp bay leaf powder
- ½ tsp ground black pepper
- ½ tsp paprika
- ¼ tsp dry mustard
- ¼ tsp cayenne pepper
- ¼ tsp allspice
- 2 pounds chicken wings

Directions:
1. Preheat your to 340 F on Air Fry function. In a bowl, mix celery salt, bay leaf powder, black pepper, paprika, dry mustard, cayenne pepper, and allspice. Coat the wings thoroughly in this mixture.
2. Arrange the wings in an even layer in the greased frying basket and fit in the baking tray. Cook the chicken until it's no longer pink around the bone, about 20 minutes. Then, increase the temperature to 380 F and cook for 6 minutes more until crispy on the outside. Serve warm.

46. Spicy Broccoli With Hot Sauce

Servings: 6
Cooking Time: 14 Minutes
Ingredients:
- Broccoli:
- 1 medium-sized head broccoli, cut into florets
- 1½ tablespoons olive oil
- 1 teaspoon shallot powder
- 1 teaspoon porcini powder
- ½ teaspoon freshly grated lemon zest
- ½ teaspoon hot paprika
- ½ teaspoon granulated garlic
- $^1/_3$ teaspoon fine sea salt
- $^1/_3$ teaspoon celery seeds
- Hot Sauce:
- ½ cup tomato sauce
- 1 tablespoon balsamic vinegar
- ½ teaspoon ground allspice

Directions:
1. In a mixing bowl, combine all the ingredients for the broccoli and toss to coat. Transfer the broccoli to the air fryer basket.
2. Put the air fryer basket on the baking pan and slide into Rack Position 2, select Air Fry, set temperature to 360ºF (182ºC), and set time to 14 minutes.
3. Meanwhile, make the hot sauce by whisking together the tomato sauce, balsamic vinegar, and allspice in a small bowl.
4. When cooking is complete, remove the broccoli from the oven and serve with the hot sauce.

47. Cajun Shrimp

Servings:3
Cooking Time: 15 Minutes
Ingredients:
- ½ pound shrimp, deveined
- ½ tsp Cajun seasoning
- Salt and black pepper to taste
- 1 tbsp olive oil

Directions:
1. Preheat on AirFry function to 390 F. In a bowl, make the marinade by mixing salt, pepper, olive oil, and seasoning. Add in the shrimp and toss to coat. Transfer the prepared shrimp to the frying basket and place in the oven. Press Start and cook for 10-12 minutes.

48. Herbed Radish Sauté(1)

Servings: 4
Cooking Time: 20 Minutes
Ingredients:
- 2 bunches red radishes; halved
- 2 tbsp. parsley; chopped.
- 2 tbsp. balsamic vinegar
- 1 tbsp. olive oil
- Salt and black pepper to taste.

Directions:
1. Take a bowl and mix the radishes with the remaining ingredients except the parsley, toss and put them in your air fryer's basket.
2. Cook at 400°F for 15 minutes, divide between plates, sprinkle the parsley on top and serve as a side dish
- **Nutrition Info:** Calories: 180; Fat: 4g; Fiber: 2g; Carbs: 3g; Protein: 5g

49. Bacon Wrapped Asparagus

Servings: 4
Cooking Time: 4
Ingredients:
- 20 spears asparagus
- 4 bacon slices
- 1 tbsp olive oil
- 1 tbsp sesame oil
- 1 tbsp brown sugar
- 1 garlic clove, crushed

Directions:
1. Preheat on Air Fry function to 380 F. In a bowl, mix the oils, sugar, and crushed garlic. Separate the asparagus into 4 bunches (5 spears in 1 bunch) and wrap each bunch with a bacon slice. Coat the bunches with the oil mixture. Place them in your Air Fryer basket and fit in the baking tray. Cook for 8 minutes, shaling once. Serve warm.

50. Spinach And Artichokes Sauté

Servings: 4
Cooking Time: 20 Minutes

Ingredients:
- 10 oz. artichoke hearts; halved
- 2 cups baby spinach
- 3 garlic cloves
- ¼ cup veggie stock
- 2 tsp. lime juice
- Salt and black pepper to taste.

Directions:
1. In a pan that fits your air fryer, mix all the ingredients, toss, introduce in the fryer and cook at 370°F for 15 minutes
2. Divide between plates and serve as a side dish.
- **Nutrition Info:** Calories: 209; Fat: 6g; Fiber: 2g; Carbs: 4g; Protein: 8g

51. Cheddar Tortilla Chips

Servings:4
Cooking Time: 20 Minutes
Ingredients:
- 1 cup flour
- Salt and black pepper to taste
- 1 tbsp golden flaxseed meal
- 2 cups shredded Cheddar cheese

Directions:
1. Melt cheddar cheese in the microwave for 1 minute. Once melted, add the flour, salt, flaxseed meal, and pepper. Mix well with a fork.
2. On a board, place the dough and knead it with hands while warm until the ingredients are well combined. Divide the dough into 2 and with a rolling pin, roll them out flat into 2 rectangles.
3. Use a pastry cutter to cut out triangle-shaped pieces and line them in a single layer on a baking dish without touching or overlapping; spray with cooking spray.
4. Select AirFry function, adjust the temperature to 380 F, and press Start. Cook for 10 minutes. Serve with tomato sauce.

52. Potato Chips With Creamy Lemon Dip

Servings:3
Cooking Time: 25 Minutes
Ingredients:
- 3 large potatoes
- 1 cup sour cream
- 2 scallions, white part minced
- 3 tbsp olive oil.
- ½ tsp lemon juice
- salt and black pepper

Directions:
1. Preheat on AirFry function to 350 F. Cut the potatoes into thin slices; do not peel them. Brush them with olive oil and season with salt and pepper. Arrange on the frying basket.

2. Press Start on the oven and cook for 20-25 minutes. Season with salt and pepper. To prepare the dip, mix together the sour cream, olive oil, scallions, lemon juice, salt, and pepper.

53. Beef Enchilada Dip

Servings: 8
Cooking Time: 10 Minutes
Ingredients:
- 2 lbs. ground beef
- ½ onion, chopped fine
- 2 cloves garlic, chopped fine
- 2 cups enchilada sauce
- 2 cups Monterrey Jack cheese, grated
- 2 tbsp. sour cream

Directions:
1. Place rack in position
2. Heat a large skillet over med-high heat. Add beef and cook until it starts to brown. Drain off fat.
3. Stir in onion and garlic and cook until tender, about 3 minutes. Stir in enchilada sauce and transfer mixture to a small casserole dish and top with cheese.
4. Set oven to convection bake on 325°F for 10 minutes. After 5 minutes, add casserole to the oven and bake 3-5 minutes until cheese is melted and mixture is heated through.
5. Serve warm topped with sour cream.
- **Nutrition Info:** Calories 414, Total Fat 22g, Saturated Fat 10g, Total Carbs 15g, Net Carbs 11g, Protein 39g, Sugar 8g, Fiber 4g, Sodium 1155mg, Potassium 635mg, Phosphorus 385mg

54. Parmesan Zucchini

Servings: 4
Cooking Time: 15 Minutes
Ingredients:
- 1 lb zucchini, sliced
- 1 garlic clove, minced
- 2 tbsp olive oil
- 1 oz parmesan cheese, grated
- 1 tsp dried mixed herbs

Directions:
1. Fit the oven with the rack in position
2. Add all ingredients except parmesan cheese into the large bowl and toss well.
3. Transfer the zucchini mixture to the baking dish.
4. Set to bake at 450 F for 20 minutes. After 5 minutes place the baking dish in the preheated oven.
5. Sprinkle parmesan cheese over zucchini and bake for 5 minutes more.
- **Nutrition Info:** Calories 103 Fat 8.7 g Carbohydrates 4.4 g Sugar 1.3 g Protein 3.7 g Cholesterol 5 mg

55. Mustard Cheddar Twists

Servings:4
Cooking Time: 45 Minutes
Ingredients:
- 2 cups cauliflower florets, steamed
- 1 egg
- 3 ½ oz oats
- 1 red onion, diced
- 1 tsp mustard
- 5 oz cheddar cheese
- Salt and black pepper to taste

Directions:
1. Place the oats in a food processor and pulse until they resemble breadcrumbs. Place the steamed florets in a cheesecloth and squeeze out the excess liquid.
2. Transfer to a large bowl. Add in the rest of the ingredients. Mix well. Take a little bit of the mixture and twist it into a straw.
3. Place on a lined baking tray and repeat with the rest of the mixture. Select AirFry function, adjust the temperature to 360 F, and press Start. Cook for 10 minutes, turn over and cook for an additional 10 minutes.

56. Sesame Sticky Chicken Wings

Servings:4
Cooking Time: 45 Minutes
Ingredients:
- 1 pound chicken wings
- 1 cup soy sauce, divided
- ½ cup brown sugar
- ½ cup apple cider vinegar
- 2 tbsp fresh ginger, minced
- 2 tbsp fresh garlic, minced
- 1 tsp finely ground black pepper
- 2 tbsp cornstarch
- 2 tbsp cold water
- 1 tsp sesame seeds

Directions:
1. In a bowl, add chicken wings and pour in a half cup of the soy sauce. Place in the fridge for 20 minutes. Then, drain and pat dry. Arrange the wings on the frying basket. Select AirFry function, adjust the temperature to 380 F, and press Start. Cook for 20-25 minutes at 380 F. Make sure you check them towards the end to avoid overcooking.
2. In a skillet and over medium heat, pour the remaining soy sauce, vinegar, sugar, ginger, garlic, and black pepper. Stir until sauce has reduced slightly, about 4 to 6 minutes.
3. Dissolve cornstarch in cold water and stir in the sauce. Cook until it thickens, about 2 minutes. Pour the sauce over the wings and sprinkle with sesame seeds to serve.

57. Buffalo Quesadillas

Servings: 8
Cooking Time: 5 Minutes

Ingredients:

- Nonstick cooking spray
- 2 cups chicken, cooked & chopped fine
- ½ cup Buffalo wing sauce
- 2 cups Monterey Jack cheese, grated
- ½ cup green onions, sliced thin
- 8 flour tortillas, 8-inch diameter
- ¼ cup blue cheese dressing

Directions:

1. Lightly spray the baking pan with cooking spray.
2. In a medium bowl, add chicken and wing sauce and toss to coat.
3. Place tortillas, one at a time on work surface. Spread ¼ of the chicken mixture over tortilla and sprinkle with cheese and onion. Top with a second tortilla and place on the baking pan.
4. Set oven to broil on 400°F for 8 minutes. After 5 minutes place baking pan in position 2. Cook quesadillas 2-3 minutes per side until toasted and cheese has melted. Repeat with remaining ingredients.
5. Cut quesadillas in wedges and serve with blue cheese dressing or other dipping sauce.

- **Nutrition Info:** Calories 376, Total Fat 20g, Saturated Fat 8g, Total Carbs 27g, Net Carbs 26g, Protein 22g, Sugar 2g, Fiber 2g, Sodium 685mg, Potassium 201mg, Phosphorus 301mg

BREAKFAST RECIPES

58. Egg & Bacon Wraps With Salsa

Servings:3
Cooking Time: 15 Minutes
Ingredients:
- 3 tortillas
- 2 previously scrambled eggs
- 3 slices bacon, cut into strips
- 3 tbsp salsa
- 3 tbsp cream cheese
- 1 cup Pepper Jack cheese, grated

Directions:
1. Preheat on AirFry function to 390 F. Spread 1 tbsp of cream cheese onto each tortilla. Divide the eggs and bacon between the tortillas evenly. Top with salsa and sprinkle some grated cheese over. Roll up the tortillas and press Start. Cook for 10 minutes. Serve.

59. Rice, Shrimp, And Spinach Frittata

Servings:4
Cooking Time: 16 Minutes
Ingredients:
- 4 eggs
- Pinch salt
- ½ cup cooked rice
- ½ cup chopped cooked shrimp
- ½ cup baby spinach
- ½ cup grated Monterey Jack cheese
- Nonstick cooking spray

Directions:
1. Spritz the baking pan with nonstick cooking spray.
2. Whisk the eggs and salt in a small bowl until frothy.
3. Place the cooked rice, shrimp, and baby spinach in the baking pan. Pour in the whisked eggs and scatter the cheese on top.
4. Slide the baking pan into Rack Position 1, select Convection Bake, set temperature to 320ºF (160ºC) and set time to 16 minutes.
5. When cooking is complete, the frittata should be golden and puffy.
6. Let the frittata cool for 5 minutes before slicing to serve.

60. Eggs In A Hole

Servings: 1
Cooking Time: 7 Minutes
Ingredients:
- 2 eggs
- 2 slices of bread
- 2 tsp butter
- Pepper and salt to taste

Directions:

1. Using a jar punch two holes in the middle of your bread slices. This is the area where you will place your eggs.
2. Preheat your fryer to 330-degree Fahrenheit for about 5 minutes. Spread a tablespoon of butter into the pan and then add bread from the slices.
3. Crack the eggs and place them at the center of the bread slices and lightly season them with salt and pepper.
4. Take out your slices and rebutter the pan with the remaining butter and fry the other part for 3 minutes.
5. Serve while hot.
- **Nutrition Info:** Calories 787 Fat 51g, Carbohydrates 60g, Proteins 22g.

61. Tator Tots Casserole

Servings: 8
Cooking Time: 30 Minutes
Ingredients:
- 8 eggs
- 28 oz tator tots
- 8 oz pepper jack cheese, shredded
- 2 green onions, sliced
- 1/4 cup milk
- 1 lb breakfast sausage, cooked
- Pepper
- Salt

Directions:
1. Fit the oven with the rack in position
2. Spray 13*9-inch baking pan with cooking spray and set aside.
3. In a bowl, whisk eggs with milk, pepper, and salt.
4. Layer sausage in a prepared baking pan then pour the egg mixture and sprinkle with half shredded cheese and green onions.
5. Add tator tots on top.
6. Set to bake at 400 F for 35 minutes. After 5 minutes place the baking pan in the preheated oven.
7. Top with remaining cheese and serve.
- **Nutrition Info:** Calories 398 Fat 31.5 g Carbohydrates 2 g Sugar 0.8 g Protein 22.1 g Cholesterol 251 mg

62. Baked Avocado With Eggs

Servings:2
Cooking Time: 9 Minutes
Ingredients:
- 1 large avocado, halved and pitted
- 2 large eggs
- 2 tomato slices, divided
- ½ cup nonfat Cottage cheese, divided
- ½ teaspoon fresh cilantro, for garnish

Directions:
1. Line the baking pan with aluminium foil.

2. Slice a thin piece from the bottom of each avocado half so they sit flat. Remove a small amount from each avocado half to make a bigger hole to hold the egg.
3. Arrange the avocado halves on the pan, hollow-side up. Break 1 egg into each half. Top each half with 1 tomato slice and ¼ cup of the Cottage cheese.
4. Slide the baking pan into Rack Position 1, select Convection Bake, set temperature to 425ºF (220ºC) and set time to 9 minutes.
5. When cooking is complete, remove the pan from the oven. Garnish with the fresh cilantro and serve.

63. Air Fryer Breakfast Frittata

Servings: 2
Cooking Time: 20 Minutes
Ingredients:
- ¼ pound breakfast sausage, fully cooked and crumbled
- 4 eggs, lightly beaten
- ½ cup Monterey Jack cheese, shredded
- 2 tablespoons red bell pepper, diced
- 1 green onion, chopped
- 1 pinch cayenne pepper

Directions:
1. Preheat the Air fryer to 365 ºF and grease a nonstick 6x2-inch cake pan.
2. Whisk together eggs with sausage, green onion, bell pepper, cheese and cayenne in a bowl.
3. Transfer the egg mixture in the prepared cake pan and place in the Air fryer.
4. Cook for about 20 minutes and serve warm.
- **Nutrition Info:** Calories: 464, Fat: 33.7g, Carbohydrates: 10.4g, Sugar: 7g, Protein: 30.4g, Sodium: 704mg

64. Feta & Tomato Tart With Olives

Servings:2
Cooking Time: 40 Minutes
Ingredients:
- 4 eggs
- ½ cup tomatoes, chopped
- 1 cup feta cheese, crumbled
- 1 tbsp fresh basil, chopped
- 1 tbsp fresh oregano, chopped
- ¼ cup Kalamata olives, pitted and chopped
- ¼ cup onions, chopped
- 2 tbsp olive oil
- ½ cup milk
- Salt and black pepper to taste

Directions:
1. Preheat on Bake function to 340 F. Brush a pie pan with olive oil. Beat the eggs along with the milk, salt, and pepper. Stir in the remaining ingredients. Pour the egg mixture

into the pan and press Start. Cook for 15-18 minutes. Serve sliced.

65. Broccoli Asparagus Frittata

Servings: 6
Cooking Time: 20 Minutes
Ingredients:
- 6 eggs
- 1/2 cup onion, diced & sautéed
- 1 cup asparagus, chopped & sautéed
- 1 cup broccoli, chopped & sautéed
- 3 bacon slices, cooked & chopped
- 1/3 cup parmesan cheese, grated
- 1/2 cup milk
- 1/2 tsp pepper
- 1 tsp salt

Directions:
1. Fit the oven with the rack in position
2. In a mixing bowl, whisk eggs with milk, cheese, pepper, and salt.
3. Add onion, asparagus, broccoli, and bacon and stir well.
4. Pour egg mixture into the greased baking dish.
5. Set to bake at 350 F for 25 minutes. After 5 minutes place the baking dish in the preheated oven.
6. Serve and enjoy.
- **Nutrition Info:** Calories 154 Fat 9.9 g Carbohydrates 4.6 g Sugar 2.4 g Protein 12.4 g Cholesterol 179 mg

66. Almond & Cinnamon Berry Oat Bars

Servings: 10
Cooking Time: 40 Minutes
Ingredients:
- 3 cups rolled oats
- ½ cup ground almonds
- ½ cup flour
- 1 tsp baking powder
- 1 tsp ground cinnamon
- 3 eggs, lightly beaten
- ½ cup canola oil
- ⅓ cup milk
- 2 tsp vanilla extract
- 2 cups mixed berries

Directions:
1. Spray the baking pan with cooking spray. In a bowl, add oats, almonds, flour, baking powder and cinnamon into and stir well. In another bowl, whisk eggs, oil, milk, and vanilla.
2. Stir the wet ingredients gently into the oat mixture. Fold in the berries. Pour the mixture in the pan and place in the toaster oven. Cook for 15-20 minutes at 350 F on Bake function until is nice and soft. Let cool and cut into bars to serve.

67. Whole-wheat Blueberry Scones

Servings: 14
Cooking Time: 20 Minutes
Ingredients:
- ½ cup low-fat buttermilk
- ¾ cup orange juice
- Zest of 1 orange
- 2¼ cups whole-wheat pastry flour
- $^1/_3$ cup agave nectar
- ¼ cup canola oil
- 1 teaspoon baking soda
- 1 teaspoon cream of tartar
- 1 cup fresh blueberries

Directions:
1. In a small bowl, stir together the buttermilk, orange juice and orange zest.
2. In a large bowl, whisk together the flour, agave nectar, canola oil, baking soda and cream of tartar.
3. Add the buttermilk mixture and blueberries to the bowl with the flour mixture. Mix gently by hand until well combined.
4. Transfer the batter onto a lightly floured baking pan. Pat into a circle about ¾ inch thick and 8 inches across. Use a knife to cut the circle into 14 wedges, cutting almost all the way through.
5. Slide the baking pan into Rack Position 1, select Convection Bake, set temperature to 375ºF (190ºC) and set time to 20 minutes.
6. When cooking is complete, remove the pan and check the scones. They should be lightly browned.
7. Let rest for 5 minutes and cut completely through the wedges before serving.

68. Thai Style Omelette

Servings: 2
Cooking Time: 10 Minutes
Ingredients:
- 3 & 1/2 oz minced Pancetta
- 2 Eggs
- 1 cup onion, diced
- 1 tablespoon fish salt

Directions:
1. Beat the eggs until it is light and fluffy. Preheat the Air fryer to 280°F.
2. In a bowl, add together all the ingredients. Pour the mixture into the air fryer tray.
3. Remove after 10 minutes or once omelet is golden brown. Cut and serve.
- **Nutrition Info:** Calories 113 Fat 8.2 g Carbohydrates 0.3 g Sugar 0.2 g Protein 5.4 g Cholesterol 18 mg

69. Meat Lover Omelet With Mozzarella

Servings: 2
Cooking Time: 20 Minutes
Ingredients:
- 1 beef sausage, chopped
- 4 slices prosciutto, chopped
- 3 oz salami, chopped
- 1 cup grated mozzarella cheese
- 4 eggs
- 1 tbsp chopped onion
- 1 tbsp ketchup

Directions:
1. Preheat on Bake function to 350 F. Whisk the eggs with ketchup in a bowl. Stir in the onion. Brown the sausage in a greased pan over medium heat for 2 minutes.
2. Combine the egg mixture, mozzarella cheese, salami, and prosciutto. Pour the egg mixture over the sausage and give it a stir. Press Start and cook in the for 15 minutes.

70. Simply Bacon

Servings: 1 Person
Cooking Time: 10 Minutes
Ingredients:
- 4 pieces of bacon

Directions:
1. Place the bacon strips on the instant vortex air fryer.
2. Cook for 10 minutes
3. at 200 degrees Celsius.
4. Check when it browns and shows to be ready. Serve.
- **Nutrition Info:** Calories 165, Fat 13g, Proteins 12 g, Carbs 0g

71. Cabbage And Mushroom Spring Rolls

Servings: 14 Spring Rolls
Cooking Time: 14 Minutes
Ingredients:
- 2 tablespoons vegetable oil
- 4 cups sliced Napa cabbage
- 5 ounces (142 g) shiitake mushrooms, diced
- 3 carrots, cut into thin matchsticks
- 1 tablespoon minced fresh ginger
- 1 tablespoon minced garlic
- 1 bunch scallions, white and light green parts only, sliced
- 2 tablespoons soy sauce
- 1 (4-ounce / 113-g) package cellophane noodles
- ¼ teaspoon cornstarch
- 1 (12-ounce / 340-g) package frozen spring roll wrappers, thawed
- Cooking spray

Directions:
1. Heat the olive oil in a nonstick skillet over medium-high heat until shimmering.
2. Add the cabbage, mushrooms, and carrots and sauté for 3 minutes or until tender.
3. Add the ginger, garlic, and scallions and sauté for 1 minutes or until fragrant.

4. Mix in the soy sauce and turn off the heat. Discard any liquid remains in the skillet and allow to cool for a few minutes.
5. Bring a pot of water to a boil, then turn off the heat and pour in the noodles. Let sit for 10 minutes or until the noodles are al dente. Transfer 1 cup of the noodles in the skillet and toss with the cooked vegetables. Reserve the remaining noodles for other use.
6. Dissolve the cornstarch in a small dish of water, then place the wrappers on a clean work surface. Dab the edges of the wrappers with cornstarch.
7. Scoop up 3 tablespoons of filling in the center of each wrapper, then fold the corner in front of you over the filling. Tuck the wrapper under the filling, then fold the corners on both sides into the center. Keep rolling to seal the wrapper. Repeat with remaining wrappers.
8. Spritz the air fryer basket with cooking spray. Arrange the wrappers in the pan and spritz with cooking spray.
9. Put the air fryer basket on the baking pan and slide into Rack Position 2, select Air Fry, set temperature to 400ºF (205ºC) and set time to 10 minutes.
10. Flip the wrappers halfway through the cooking time.
11. When cooking is complete, the wrappers will be golden brown.
12. Serve immediately.

72. Salsa Verde Golden Chicken Empanadas

Servings: 12 Empanadas
Cooking Time: 12 Minutes
Ingredients:
- 1 cup boneless, skinless rotisserie chicken breast meat, chopped finely
- ¼ cup salsa verde
- $^2/_3$ cup shredded Cheddar cheese
- 1 teaspoon ground cumin
- 1 teaspoon ground black pepper
- 2 purchased refrigerated pie crusts, from a minimum 14.1-ounce (400 g) box
- 1 large egg
- 2 tablespoons water
- Cooking spray

Directions:
1. Spritz the air fryer basket with cooking spray. Set aside.
2. Combine the chicken meat, salsa verde, Cheddar, cumin, and black pepper in a large bowl. Stir to mix well. Set aside.
3. Unfold the pie crusts on a clean work surface, then use a large cookie cutter to cut out 3½-inch circles as much as possible.

4. Roll the remaining crusts to a ball and flatten into a circle which has the same thickness of the original crust. Cut out more 3½-inch circles until you have 12 circles in total.
5. Make the empanadas: Divide the chicken mixture in the middle of each circle, about 1½ tablespoons each. Dab the edges of the circle with water. Fold the circle in half over the filling to shape like a half-moon and press to seal, or you can press with a fork.
6. Whisk the egg with water in a small bowl.
7. Arrange the empanadas in the pan and spritz with cooking spray. Brush with whisked egg.
8. Put the air fryer basket on the baking pan and slide into Rack Position 2, select Air Fry, set temperature to 350ºF (180ºC) and set time to 12 minutes.
9. Flip the empanadas halfway through the cooking time.
10. When cooking is complete, the empanadas will be golden and crispy.
11. Serve immediately.

73. Wheat &seed Bread

Servings: 4
Cooking Time: 18 Minutes
Ingredients:
- 31/2 ounces of flour
- 1 tsp. of yeast
- 1 tsp. of salt
- 3 &1/2 ounces of wheat flour ¼ cup of pumpkin seeds

Directions:
1. Mix the wheat flour, yeast, salt, seeds and the plain flour together in a large bowl. Stir in ¾ cup of lukewarm water and keep stirring until dough becomes soft.
2. Knead for another 5 minutes until the dough becomes elastic and smooth. Mold into a ball and cover with a plastic bag. Set aside for 30 minutes for it to rise.
3. Heat your air fryer to 392°F.
4. Transfer the dough into a small pizza pan and place in the air fryer. Bake for 18 minutes until golden. Remove and place on a wire rack to cool.
- **Nutrition Info:** Calories 116 Fat 9.4 g Carbohydrates 0.3 g Sugar 0.2 g Protein 6 g Cholesterol 21 mg

74. Easy Breakfast Bake

Servings: 6
Cooking Time: 45 Minutes
Ingredients:
- 10 eggs
- 10 bacon sliced, cooked, and crumbled
- 2 tomatoes, sliced
- 1 tbsp butter

- 3 cups baby spinach, chopped
- 1/2 tsp salt

Directions:
1. Fit the oven with the rack in position
2. Melt butter in a pan.
3. Add spinach and cook until spinach wilted.
4. Whisk eggs and salt in a bowl. Add spinach and whisk well.
5. Pour egg mixture into the greased 9-inch baking dish. Top with bacon and tomatoes
6. Set to bake at 350 F for 50 minutes, after 5 minutes, place the baking dish in the oven.
7. Serve and enjoy.
- **Nutrition Info:** Calories 266 Fat 21 g Carbohydrates 2.7 g Sugar 1.7 g Protein 18.4 g Cholesterol 303 mg

75. Italian Sandwich

Servings:1
Cooking Time: 7 Minutes
Ingredients:
- 2 bread slices
- 4 tomato slices
- 4 mozzarella cheese slices
- 1 tbsp olive oil
- 1 tbsp fresh basil, chopped
- Salt and black pepper to taste

Directions:
1. Preheat on Toast function to 350 F. Place the bread slices in the toaster oven and toast for 5 minutes. Arrange two tomato slices on each bread slice. Season with salt and pepper.
2. Top each slice with 2 mozzarella slices. Return to the oven and cook for 1 more minute. Drizzle the caprese toasts with olive oil and top with chopped basil.

76. Peanut Butter And Jelly Banana Boats

Servings: 1
Cooking Time: 15 Minutes
Ingredients:
- 1 banana
- 1/4 cup peanut butter
- 1/4 cup jelly
- 1 tablespoon granola

Directions:
1. Start by preheating toaster oven to 350°F.
2. Slice banana lengthwise and separate slightly.
3. Spread peanut butter and jelly in the gap.
4. Sprinkle granola over the entire banana.
5. Bake for 15 minutes.
- **Nutrition Info:** Calories: 724, Sodium: 327 mg, Dietary Fiber: 9.2 g, Total Fat: 36.6 g, Total Carbs: 102.9 g, Protein: 20.0 g.

77. Baked Apple Breakfast Oats

Servings: 1

Cooking Time: 15 Minutes
Ingredients:
- 1/3 cup vanilla Greek yogurt
- 1/3 cup rolled oats
- 1 apple
- 1 tablespoon peanut butter

Directions:
1. Preheat toaster oven to 400°F and set it on the warm setting.
2. Cut apples into chunks approximately 1/2-inch-thick.
3. Place apples in an oven-safe dish with some space between each chunk and sprinkle with cinnamon.
4. Bake in the oven for 12 minutes.
5. Combine yogurt and oats in a bowl.
6. Remove the apples from the oven and combine with the yogurt.
7. Top with peanut butter for a delicious and high-protein breakfast.
- **Nutrition Info:** Calories: 350, Sodium: 134 mg, Dietary Fiber: 8.1 g, Total Fat: 11.2 g, Total Carbs: 52.5 g, Protein: 12.7 g.

78. Apple Cinnamon Oat Muffins

Servings: 12
Cooking Time: 15 Minutes
Ingredients:
- 1 egg
- 1 apple, peel & dice
- 1 tsp cinnamon
- 1/2 cup milk
- 2 bananas, mashed
- 2 cups rolled oats
- 1 tsp baking powder
- Pinch of salt

Directions:
1. Fit the oven with the rack in position
2. Line the muffin tray with cupcake liners and set aside.
3. In a mixing bowl, whisk the egg with cinnamon, baking powder, milk, oats, bananas, and salt.
4. Add apple and stir well.
5. Pour mixture into the prepared muffin tray.
6. Set to bake at 375 F for 20 minutes. After 5 minutes place the muffin tray in the preheated oven.
7. Serve and enjoy.
- **Nutrition Info:** Calories 90 Fat 1.6 g Carbohydrates 17.2 g Sugar 5 g Protein 2.9 g Cholesterol 14 mg

79. Mexican Flavor Chicken Burgers

Servings:6 To 8
Cooking Time: 20 Minutes
Ingredients:
- 4 skinless and boneless chicken breasts

- 1 small head of cauliflower, sliced into florets
- 1 jalapeño pepper
- 3 tablespoons smoked paprika
- 1 tablespoon thyme
- 1 tablespoon oregano
- 1 tablespoon mustard powder
- 1 teaspoon cayenne pepper
- 1 egg
- Salt and ground black pepper, to taste
- 2 tomatoes, sliced
- 2 lettuce leaves, chopped
- 6 to 8 brioche buns, sliced lengthwise
- ¾ cup taco sauce
- Cooking spray

Directions:
1. Spritz the air fryer basket with cooking spray. Set aside.
2. In a blender, add the cauliflower florets, jalapeño pepper, paprika, thyme, oregano, mustard powder and cayenne pepper and blend until the mixture has a texture similar to bread crumbs.
3. Transfer ¾ of the cauliflower mixture to a medium bowl and set aside. Beat the egg in a different bowl and set aside.
4. Add the chicken breasts to the blender with remaining cauliflower mixture. Sprinkle with salt and pepper. Blend until finely chopped and well mixed.
5. Remove the mixture from the blender and form into 6 to 8 patties. One by one, dredge each patty in the reserved cauliflower mixture, then into the egg. Dip them in the cauliflower mixture again for additional coating.
6. Place the coated patties into the pan and spritz with cooking spray.
7. Put the air fryer basket on the baking pan and slide into Rack Position 2, select Air Fry, set temperature to 350ºF (180ºC) and set time to 20 minutes.
8. Flip the patties halfway through the cooking time.
9. When cooking is complete, the patties should be golden and crispy.
10. Transfer the patties to a clean work surface and assemble with the buns, tomato slices, chopped lettuce leaves and taco sauce to make burgers. Serve and enjoy.

80. Potato Egg Casserole

Servings: 6
Cooking Time: 35 Minutes
Ingredients:
- 5 eggs
- 2 medium potatoes, cut into 1/2-inch cubes
- 1 green bell pepper, diced
- 1 small onion, chopped

- 1 tbsp olive oil
- 1/2 cup cheddar cheese, shredded
- 3/4 tsp pepper
- 3/4 tsp salt

Directions:
1. Fit the oven with the rack in position
2. Spray 9*9-inch casserole dish with cooking spray and set aside.
3. Heat oil in a pan over medium heat.
4. Add onion and sauté for 1 minute. Add potatoes, bell peppers, 1/2 tsp pepper, and 1/2 tsp salt and sauté for 4 minutes.
5. Transfer sautéed vegetables to the prepared casserole dish and spread evenly.
6. In a bowl, whisk eggs with remaining pepper and salt.
7. Pour egg mixture over sautéed vegetables in a casserole dish. Sprinkle cheese on top.
8. Set to bake at 350 F for 40 minutes. After 5 minutes place the casserole dish in the preheated oven.
9. Serve and enjoy.
- **Nutrition Info:** Calories 171 Fat 9.2 g Carbohydrates 14.3 g Sugar 2.6 g Protein 8.5 g Cholesterol 146 mg

81. Crispy Chicken Egg Rolls

Servings:4
Cooking Time: 23 To 24 Minutes
Ingredients:
- 1 pound (454 g) ground chicken
- 2 teaspoons olive oil
- 2 garlic cloves, minced
- 1 teaspoon grated fresh ginger
- 2 cups white cabbage, shredded
- 1 onion, chopped
- ¼ cup soy sauce
- 8 egg roll wrappers
- 1 egg, beaten
- Cooking spray

Directions:
1. Spritz the air fryer basket with cooking spray.
2. Heat olive oil in a saucepan over medium heat. Sauté the garlic and ginger in the olive oil for 1 minute, or until fragrant. Add the ground chicken to the saucepan. Sauté for 5 minutes, or until the chicken is cooked through. Add the cabbage, onion and soy sauce and sauté for 5 to 6 minutes, or until the vegetables become soft. Remove the saucepan from the heat.
3. Unfold the egg roll wrappers on a clean work surface. Divide the chicken mixture among the wrappers and brush the edges of the wrappers with the beaten egg. Tightly roll up the egg rolls, enclosing the filling. Arrange the rolls in the pan.

4. Put the air fryer basket on the baking pan and slide into Rack Position 2, select Air Fry, set temperature to 370ºF (188ºC) and set time to 12 minutes.
5. Flip the rolls halfway through the cooking time.
6. When cooked, the rolls will be crispy and golden brown.
7. Transfer to a platter and let cool for 5 minutes before serving.

82. Berry Breakfast Oatmeal

Servings: 4
Cooking Time: 20 Minutes
Ingredients:
- 1 egg
- 2 cups old fashioned oats
- 1 cup blueberries
- 1/4 cup maple syrup
- 1 1/2 cups milk
- 1/2 cup blackberries
- 1/2 cup strawberries, sliced
- 1 1/2 tsp baking powder
- 1/2 tsp salt

Directions:
1. Fit the oven with the rack in position
2. In a bowl, mix together oats, salt, and baking powder.
3. Add vanilla, egg, maple syrup, and milk and stir well. Add berries and fold well.
4. Pour mixture into the greased baking dish.
5. Set to bake at 375 F for 25 minutes. After 5 minutes place the baking dish in the preheated oven.
6. Serve and enjoy.
- **Nutrition Info:** Calories 461 Fat 8.4 g Carbohydrates 80.7 g Sugar 23.4 g Protein 15 g Cholesterol 48 mg

83. Banana Cake With Peanut Butter

Servings:2
Cooking Time: 35 Minutes
Ingredients:
- 1 cup + 1 tbsp flour
- 1 tsp baking powder
- ⅓ cup sugar
- 2 bananas, mashed
- ¼ cup vegetable oil
- 1 egg, beaten
- 1 tsp vanilla extract
- ¾ cup chopped walnuts
- ¼ tsp salt
- 2 tbsp peanut butter
- 2 tbsp sour cream

Directions:
1. Preheat on AirFry function to 330 F. In a bowl, combine flour, salt, and baking powder In another bowl, combine bananas, oil, egg, peanut butter, vanilla, sugar, and sour cream.
2. Gently mix the both mixtures. Stir in the chopped walnuts. Pour the batter into a greased baking dish and press Start. Cook for 25 minutes. Serve chilled.

84. Cinnamon-orange Toast

Servings: 6
Cooking Time: 15 Minutes
Ingredients:
- 12 slices bread
- ½ cup sugar
- 1 stick butter
- 1½ tbsp vanilla extract
- 1½ tbsp cinnamon
- 2 oranges, zested

Directions:
1. Mix butter, sugar, and vanilla extract and microwave for 30 seconds until everything melts. Add in orange zest. Pour the mixture over bread slices. Lay the bread slices in your Air Fryer pan and cook for 5 minutes at 400 F on Toast function. Serve with berry sauce.

85. Cinnamon & Vanilla Toast

Servings:6
Cooking Time: 10 Minutes
Ingredients:
- 12 bread slices
- ½ cup sugar
- 1 ½ tsp cinnamon
- 1 stick of butter, softened
- 1 tsp vanilla extract

Directions:
1. Preheat on Toast function to 300 F. Combine all ingredients, except the bread, in a bowl. Spread the buttery cinnamon mixture onto the bread slices. Place the bread slices in the oven and press Start. Cook for 8 minutes. Serve.

86. Poppy Seed Muffins

Servings: 12
Cooking Time: 20 Minutes
Ingredients:
- 3 tbsp poppy seeds
- 1 tsp vanilla
- 8 tbsp maple syrup
- 2 tbsp lemon zest
- 6 tbsp lemon juice
- 4/5 cup almond milk
- 1/4 cup butter, melted
- 1/4 tsp baking soda
- 2 tsp baking powder
- 1 1/4 cups flour
- 1 1/4 cups almond flour
- Pinch of salt

Directions:

1. Fit the oven with the rack in position
2. Line 12-cups muffin tin with cupcake liners and set aside.
3. In a large bowl, mix together melted butter, milk, lemon zest, vanilla, lemon juice, poppy seeds, maple syrup, and almond flour.
4. Add flour, baking soda, and baking powder. Stir until well combined.
5. Pour batter into the prepared muffin tin.
6. Set to bake at 350 F for 25 minutes, after 5 minutes, place the muffin tin in the oven.
7. Serve and enjoy.

- **Nutrition Info:** Calories 239 Fat 14.4 g Carbohydrates 23.6 g Sugar 9.1 g Protein 4.7 g Cholesterol 10 mg

87. Feta & Egg Rolls

Servings:4
Cooking Time: 50 Minutes
Ingredients:

- 1 cup feta cheese, crumbled
- 2 tbsp olive oil
- 4 eggs, beaten
- 5 sheets frozen filo pastry, thawed

Directions:

1. Gently unroll the filo sheets. Brush them with olive oil. In a bowl, mix feta cheese and eggs, and parsley. Divide the feta mixture between the sheets.
2. Using your fingers, roll them upwards like a long sausage. Place the rolls in a greased baking dish and cook in the oven for 30-35 minutes at 360 F on Bake function. Serve warm.

88. Kale Egg Muffins

Servings: 12
Cooking Time: 35 Minutes
Ingredients:

- 10 eggs
- 1/4 cup kale, chopped
- 1/4 cup sausage, sliced
- 1/4 cup sun-dried tomatoes, chopped
- 1 cup almond milk
- Pepper
- Salt

Directions:

1. Fit the oven with the rack in position
2. Spray 12-cups muffin tin with cooking spray and set aside.
3. In a large bowl, add all ingredients and whisk until well combined.
4. Pour egg mixture into the greased muffin tin.
5. Set to bake at 350 F for 40 minutes, after 5 minutes, place the muffin tin in the oven.
6. Serve and enjoy.

- **Nutrition Info:** Calories 102 Fat 8.6 g Carbohydrates 1.7 g Sugar 1.1 g Protein 5.3 g Cholesterol 137 mg

89. Egg And Avocado Burrito

Servings:4
Cooking Time: 4 Minutes
Ingredients:

- 4 low-sodium whole-wheat flour tortillas
- Filling:
- 1 hard-boiled egg, chopped
- 2 hard-boiled egg whites, chopped
- 1 ripe avocado, peeled, pitted, and chopped
- 1 red bell pepper, chopped
- 1 (1.2-ounce / 34-g) slice low-sodium, low-fat American cheese, torn into pieces
- 3 tablespoons low-sodium salsa, plus additional for serving (optional)
- Special Equipment:
- 4 toothpicks (optional), soaked in water for at least 30 minutes

Directions:

1. Make the filling: Combine the egg, egg whites, avocado, red bell pepper, cheese, and salsa in a medium bowl and stir until blended.
2. Assemble the burritos: Arrange the tortillas on a clean work surface and place ¼ of the prepared filling in the middle of each tortilla, leaving about 1½-inch on each end unfilled. Fold in the opposite sides of each tortilla and roll up. Secure with toothpicks through the center, if needed.
3. Transfer the burritos to the air fryer basket.
4. Put the air fryer basket on the baking pan and slide into Rack Position 2, select Air Fry, set temperature to 390ºF (199ºC) and set time to 4 minutes.
5. When cooking is complete, the burritos should be crisp and golden brown.
6. Allow to cool for 5 minutes and serve with salsa, if desired.

90. Vanilla Brownies With White Chocolate & Walnuts

Servings: 4
Cooking Time: 35 Minutes
Ingredients:

- 6 oz dark chocolate, chopped
- 6 oz butter
- ¾ cup white sugar
- 3 eggs, beaten
- 2 tsp vanilla extract
- ¾ cup flour
- ¼ cup cocoa powder
- 1 cup chopped walnuts
- 1 cup white chocolate chips

Directions:

1. Line a baking pan with parchment paper. In a saucepan, melt chocolate and butter over low heat. Do not stop stirring until you obtain a smooth mixture. Let cool slightly and whisk in eggs and vanilla. Sift flour and cocoa and stir to mix well.
2. Sprinkle the walnuts over and add the white chocolate into the batter. Pour the batter into the pan and cook for 20 minutes in the oven at 350 F on Bake function. Serve chilled with raspberry syrup and ice cream.

91. Breakfast Cheese Sandwiches

Servings:2
Cooking Time: 8 Minutes
Ingredients:
- 1 teaspoon butter, softened
- 4 slices bread
- 4 slices smoked country ham
- 4 slices Cheddar cheese
- 4 thick slices tomato

Directions:
1. Spoon ½ teaspoon of butter onto one side of 2 slices of bread and spread it all over.
2. Assemble the sandwiches: Top each of 2 slices of unbuttered bread with 2 slices of ham, 2 slices of cheese, and 2 slices of tomato. Place the remaining 2 slices of bread on top, butter-side up.
3. Lay the sandwiches in the baking pan, buttered side down.
4. Slide the baking pan into Rack Position 1, select Convection Bake, set temperature to 370ºF (188ºC), and set time to 8 minutes.
5. Flip the sandwiches halfway through the cooking time.
6. When cooking is complete, the sandwiches should be golden brown on both sides and the cheese should be melted. Remove from the oven. Allow to cool for 5 minutes before slicing to serve.

92. Cinnamon French Toasts

Servings: 2
Cooking Time: 5 Minutes
Ingredients:
- 2 eggs
- ¼ cup whole milk
- 3 tablespoons sugar
- 2 teaspoons olive oil
- 1/8 teaspoon vanilla extract
- 1/8 teaspoon ground cinnamon
- 4 bread slices

Directions:
1. In a large bowl, mix together all the ingredients except bread slices.
2. Coat the bread slices with egg mixture evenly.

3. Press "Power Button" of Air Fry Oven and turn the dial to select the "Air Fry" mode.
4. Press the Time button and again turn the dial to set the cooking time to 6 minutes.
5. Now push the Temp button and rotate the dial to set the temperature at 390 degrees F.
6. Press "Start/Pause" button to start.
7. When the unit beeps to show that it is preheated, open the lid and lightly, grease the sheet pan.
8. Arrange the bread slices into "Air Fry Basket" and insert in the oven.
9. Flip the bread slices once halfway through.
10. Serve warm.
- **Nutrition Info:** Calories: 238 Cal Total Fat: 10.6 g Saturated Fat: 2.7 g Cholesterol: 167 mg Sodium: 122 mg Total Carbs: 20.8 g Fiber: 0.5 g Sugar: 0.9 g Protein: 7.9 g

93. Congee With Eggs With Fresh Chives

Servings:x
Cooking Time:x
Ingredients:
- 3 cups water
- 1-2 tsp hot chili oil or sesame oil
- ½ tsp kosher salt
- 2 eggs
- 1 Tbsp coarsely chopped fresh cilantro
- 1 Tbsp minced fresh chives

Directions:
1. Place the rice in a strainer and rinse well.
2. Add the rice, water, and salt to oven and cover. Place over medium-high heat and bring to a boil. As soon as the water boils, reduce the heat to low and stir the mixture. Cover and simmer for 45 minutes. After 45 minutes, the rice should be very soft and the porridge should have a silky consistency. If not, cook for another 10 minutes or so.
3. While the porridge cooks, whisk together the two eggs in a small bowl.
4. When the rice is cooked, pour the egg into the porridge in a thin stream. If you want a custardy texture, whisk the mixture quickly while you pour in the egg. If you prefer ribbons of egg, stir more slowly.
5. Cook for a minute or two or until the egg is done.
6. Stir in the cilantro and chives, and drizzle over the oil.

94. Cauliflower Tater Tots With Cheddar Cheese

Servings:6
Cooking Time: 35 Minutes
Ingredients:
- 2 lb cauliflower florets, steamed
- 5 oz cheddar cheese, grated
- 1 onion, diced

- 1 cup breadcrumbs
- 1 egg, beaten
- 1 tsp fresh parsley, chopped
- 1 tsp fresh oregano, chopped
- 1 tsp chives, chopped
- 1 tsp garlic powder
- Salt and black pepper to taste

Directions:
1. Mash the cauliflower and place it in a large bowl. Add in the onion, parsley, oregano, chives, garlic powder, cheddar cheese, salt, and pepper. Mix well and form 12 balls out of the mixture.
2. Line a baking sheet with parchment paper. Dip half of the tater tots into the egg and then coat with breadcrumbs. Arrange them on the baking sheet and cook in the preheated oven at 350 F for 15 minutes on AirFry function. Serve.

95. Moist Orange Bread Loaf

Servings: 10
Cooking Time: 50 Minutes
Ingredients:
- 4 eggs
- 4 oz butter, softened
- 1 cup of orange juice
- 1 orange zest, grated
- 1 cup of sugar
- 2 tsp baking powder
- 2 cups all-purpose flour
- 1 tsp vanilla

Directions:
1. Fit the oven with the rack in position
2. In a large bowl, whisk eggs and sugar until creamy.
3. Whisk in vanilla, butter, orange juice, and orange zest.
4. Add flour and baking powder and mix until combined.
5. Pour batter into the greased 9*5-inch loaf pan.
6. Set to bake at 350 F for 55 minutes, after 5 minutes, place the loaf pan in the oven.
7. Slice and serve.
- **Nutrition Info:** Calories 286 Fat 11.3 g Carbohydrates 42.5 g Sugar 22.4 g Protein 5.1 gCholesterol 90 mg

96. Ultimate Breakfast Sandwich

Servings: 2
Cooking Time: 5 Minutes
Ingredients:
- 2 English muffins
- 2 eggs
- 2 slices aged yellow cheddar
- 2 large spicy pork sausage patties
- Softened butter

Directions:

1. Start by setting toaster oven to toast and warming up a non-stick pan.
2. Add sausages to pan and butter the insides of the muffins.
3. While the sausages cook, put the muffins in the toaster oven to toast until crispy brown, about 5–7 minutes.
4. Set the sausages aside and add eggs to the skillet.
5. Let the whites set, then carefully flip the eggs to keep the yolks intact.
6. Turn off the heat and add cheese and sausage to the top of the eggs. This will allow everything to melt together but leave the yolks with the perfect consistency.
7. Add the mixture to the muffin and enjoy the perfect breakfast.
- **Nutrition Info:** Calories: 332, Sodium: 677 mg, Dietary Fiber: 2.0 g, Total Fat: 14.9 g, Total Carbs: 26.1 g, Protein: 22.7 g.

97. Pigs In A Blanket

Servings: 6
Cooking Time: 25 Minutes
Ingredients:
- 12 breakfast sausage links, cooked
- 6 eggs, scrambled
- ½ cup sharp cheddar cheese, grated
- ¾ cup Southwest hash browns, thawed
- 2 tubes French bread loaf, refrigerated

Directions:
1. Spray the baking pan with cooking spray.
2. Open up can of bread loaf. Divide the dough in half.
3. On a lightly floured surface, roll one half into a 5x12-inch rectangle.
4. Place 3 sausage links along the dough, leaving room in between. Cut dough into 3 equal pieces.
5. Top each sausage with a tablespoon of hash browns, tablespoon of egg, and a sprinkling of cheese. Roll up and seal the edges. Place seam side down on prepared pan. Repeat with remaining dough and filling ingredients.
6. Set oven to convection bake at 325°F for 30 minutes. After 5 minutes, place the pan in position 1 of the oven. Bake for 25 minutes, or until bread is golden brown and cooked through.
7. Let cool on wire rack 5 minutes before serving.
- **Nutrition Info:** Calories 718, Total Fat 14g, Saturated Fat 5g, Total Carbs 74g, Net Carbs 71g, Protein 24g, Sugar 7g, Fiber 3g, Sodium 1115mg, Potassium 321mg, Phosphorus 261mg

98. Beans And Pork Mix

Servings: 4

Cooking Time: 20 Minutes
Ingredients:
- 1-pound pork stew meat, ground
- 1 red onion, chopped
- 1 tablespoon olive oil
- 1 cup canned kidney beans, drained and rinsed
- 1 teaspoon chili powder
- Salt and black pepper to the taste
- ¼ teaspoon cumin, ground

Directions:
1. Heat up your air fryer at 360 degrees F, add the meat and the onion and cook for 5 minutes.
2. Add the beans and the rest of the ingredients, toss and cook for 15 minutes more.
3. Divide everything into bowls and serve for breakfast.
- **Nutrition Info:** calories 203, fat 4, fiber 6, carbs 12, protein 4

99. Classic Bacon & Egg English Muffin

Servings: 1
Cooking Time: 15 Minutes
Ingredients:
- 1 egg
- 1 English muffin
- 2 slices of bacon
- Salt and black pepper to taste

Directions:
1. Preheat on Bake function to 395 F. Crack the egg into a ramekin. Place the English muffin, egg ramekin, and bacon in a baking pan. Cook for 9 minutes. Let cool slightly so you can assemble the sandwich. Cut the muffin in half. Place the egg on one half and season with salt and pepper. Arrange the bacon on top. Top with the other muffin half.

100.Ham And Egg Toast Cups

Servings: 2
Cooking Time: 5 Minutes
Ingredients:
- 2 eggs
- 2 slices of ham
- 2 tablespoons butter
- Cheddar cheese, for topping
- Salt, to taste
- Black pepper, to taste

Directions:
1. Preheat the Air fryer to 400-degree F and grease both ramekins with melted butter.
2. Place each ham slice in the greased ramekins and crack each egg over ham slices.
3. Sprinkle with salt, black pepper and cheddar cheese and transfer into the Air fryer basket.

4. Cook for about 5 minutes and remove the ramekins from the basket.
5. Serve warm.
- **Nutrition Info:** Calories: 202, Fat: 13.7g, Carbs: 7.4g, Sugar: 3.3g, Protein: 10.2g, Sodium: 203mg

101.Healthy Squash

Servings: 4
Cooking Time: 25 Minutes
Ingredients:
- 2 lbs yellow squash, cut into half-moons
- 1 tsp Italian seasoning
- ¼ tsp pepper
- 1 tbsp olive oil
- ¼ tsp salt

Directions:
1. Add all ingredients into the large bowl and toss well.
2. Preheat the air fryer to 400 F.
3. Add squash mixture into the air fryer basket and cook for 10 minutes.
4. Shake basket and cook for another 10 minutes.
5. Shake once again and cook for 5 minutes more.
- **Nutrition Info:** Calories 70, Fat 4 g, Carbohydrates 7 g, Sugar 4 g, Protein 2 g, Cholesterol 1 mg

102.Caprese Sourdough Sandwich

Servings:2
Cooking Time: 25 Minutes
Ingredients:
- 4 sourdough bread slices
- 2 tbsp mayonnaise
- 2 slices ham
- 2 lettuce leaves
- 1 tomato, sliced
- 2 mozzarella cheese slices
- Salt and black pepper to taste

Directions:
1. On a clean board, lay the sourdough slices and spread with mayonnaise. Top 2 of the slices with ham, lettuce, tomato and mozzarella. Season with salt and pepper. Top with the remaining two slices to form two sandwiches. Spray with oil and transfer to the frying basket. Cook in the preheated oven for 14 minutes at 340 F on Bake function.

103.Egg Ham Casserole

Servings: 2
Cooking Time: 20 Minutes
Ingredients:
- 5 eggs, lightly beaten
- 1 slice bread, cut into pieces
- 1/3 cup ham, diced

- 1 tbsp pimento, diced
- 1/2 cup cheddar cheese, shredded
- 1/3 cup heavy cream
- 2 green onion, chopped
- 1/4 tsp black pepper
- 1/4 tsp salt

Directions:
1. Fit the oven with the rack in position
2. Add bread pieces to the bottom of the greased casserole dish.
3. In a bowl, whisk eggs with heavy cream, pimento, green onion, pepper, and salt.
4. Pour egg mixture over bread.
5. Sprinkle ham and cheese over egg mixture.
6. Set to bake at 350 F for 25 minutes. After 5 minutes place the casserole dish in the preheated oven.
7. Serve and enjoy.
- **Nutrition Info:** Calories 413 Fat 30 g Carbohydrates 10.7 g Sugar 4.6 g Protein 26.3 g Cholesterol 479 mg

104. Lemon Cupcakes With Orange Frosting

Servings:4
Cooking Time: 30 Minutes
Ingredients:
- Orange Frosting:
- 1 cup plain yogurt
- 2 tbsp sugar
- 1 orange, juiced and juiced
- 1 cup cream cheese
- Cupcake:
- 2 lemons, quartered and seeded
- ½ cup flour + extra for basing
- ¼ tsp salt
- 2 tbsp sugar
- 1 tsp baking powder
- 1 tsp vanilla extract
- 2 eggs
- ½ cup softened butter
- 2 tbsp milk

Directions:
1. In a bowl, mix the yogurt and cream cheese. Stir in the orange juice and zest. Gradually add the sugar while stirring until smooth. Make sure the frost is not runny. Set aside.
2. Place the lemon quarters in a food processor and process until pureed. Add in baking powder, softened butter, milk, eggs, vanilla extract, sugar, and salt. Process again until smooth.
3. Preheat on Bake function to 400 F. Flour the bottom of 8 cupcake cases and spoon the batter into the cases ¾ way up. Place them in a baking tray and press Start. Bake for 20 minutes. Remove and let cool. Design the cupcakes with the frosting to serve.

105. Egg English Muffin With Bacon

Servings:1
Cooking Time: 10 Minutes
Ingredients:
- 1 egg
- 1 English muffin
- 2 slices of bacon
- Salt and black pepper to taste

Directions:
1. Preheat on Bake function to 395 F. Crack the egg into a ramekin. Place the muffin, egg and bacon in the oven. Cook for 9 minutes. Let cool slightly so you can assemble the sandwich.
2. Cut the muffin in half. Place the egg on one half and season with salt and pepper. Arrange the bacon on top. Top with the other muffin half.

106. Caprese Sandwich With Sourdough Bread

Servings: 2
Cooking Time: 15 Minutes
Ingredients:
- 4 slices sourdough bread
- 2 tbsp mayonnaise
- 2 slices ham
- 2 lettuce leaves
- 1 tomato, sliced
- 2 slices mozzarella cheese
- Salt and black pepper to taste

Directions:
1. On a clean board, lay the sourdough slices and spread with mayonnaise. Top 2 of the slices with ham, lettuce, tomato, and mozzarella cheese. Season with salt and pepper.
2. Top with the remaining two slices to form two sandwiches. Spray with oil and transfer to the Air Fryer basket. Fit in the baking tray and cook for 10 minutes at 350 F on Bake function, flipping once halfway through cooking. Serve hot.

107. Whole-wheat Muffins With Blueberries

Servings: 8 Muffins
Cooking Time: 25 Minutes
Ingredients:
- ½ cup unsweetened applesauce
- ½ cup plant-based milk
- ½ cup maple syrup
- 1 teaspoon vanilla extract
- 2 cups whole-wheat flour
- ½ teaspoon baking soda
- 1 cup blueberries
- Cooking spray

Directions:

1. Spritz a 8-cup muffin pan with cooking spray.
2. In a large bowl, stir together the applesauce, milk, maple syrup and vanilla extract. Whisk in the flour and baking soda until no dry flour is left and the batter is smooth. Gently mix in the blueberries until they are evenly distributed throughout the batter.
3. Spoon the batter into the muffin cups, three-quarters full.
4. Put the muffin pan into Rack Position 1, select Convection Bake, set temperature to 375ºF (190ºC) and set time to 25 minutes.
5. When cooking is complete, remove from the oven and check the muffins. You can stick a knife into the center of a muffin and it should come out clean.
6. Let rest for 5 minutes before serving.

108.Blueberry Cake

Servings:8
Cooking Time: 10 Minutes
Ingredients:
- 1½ cups Bisquick
- ¼ cup granulated sugar
- 2 large eggs, beaten
- ¾ cup whole milk
- 1 teaspoon vanilla extract
- ½ teaspoon lemon zest
- Cooking spray
- 2 cups blueberries

Directions:
1. Stir together the Bisquick and sugar in a medium bowl. Stir together the eggs, milk, vanilla and lemon zest. Add the wet ingredients to the dry ingredients and stir until well combined.
2. Spritz the baking pan with cooking spray and line with parchment paper, pressing it into place. Spray the parchment paper with cooking spray. Pour the batter into the pan and spread it out evenly. Sprinkle the blueberries evenly over the top.
3. Slide the baking pan into Rack Position 1, select Convection Bake, set temperature to 375ºF (190ºC) and set time to 10 minutes.
4. When cooking is complete, the cake should be pulling away from the edges of the pan and the top should be just starting to turn golden brown.
5. Let the cake rest for a minute before cutting into 16 squares. Serve immediately.

109.Air Fried Cream Cheese Wontons

Servings:4
Cooking Time: 6 Minutes
Ingredients:
- 2 ounces (57 g) cream cheese, softened
- 1 tablespoon sugar
- 16 square wonton wrappers
- Cooking spray

Directions:
1. Spritz the air fryer basket with cooking spray.
2. In a mixing bowl, stir together the cream cheese and sugar until well mixed. Prepare a small bowl of water alongside.
3. On a clean work surface, lay the wonton wrappers. Scoop ¼ teaspoon of cream cheese in the center of each wonton wrapper. Dab the water over the wrapper edges. Fold each wonton wrapper diagonally in half over the filling to form a triangle.
4. Arrange the wontons in the pan. Spritz the wontons with cooking spray.
5. Put the air fryer basket on the baking pan and slide into Rack Position 2, select Air Fry, set temperature to 350ºF (180ºC) and set time to 6 minutes.
6. Flip the wontons halfway through the cooking time.
7. When cooking is complete, the wontons will be golden brown and crispy.
8. Divide the wontons among four plates. Let rest for 5 minutes before serving.

110.Ham And Cheese Bagel Sandwiches

Servings: 2
Cooking Time: 5 Minutes
Ingredients:
- 2 bagels
- 4 teaspoons honey mustard
- 4 slices cooked honey ham
- 4 slices Swiss cheese

Directions:
1. Start by preheating toaster oven to 400°F.
2. Spread honey mustard on each half of the bagel.
3. Add ham and cheese and close the bagel.
4. Bake the sandwich until the cheese is fully melted, approximately 5 minutes.
- **Nutrition Info:** Calories: 588, Sodium: 1450 mg, Dietary Fiber: 2.3 g, Total Fat: 20.1 g, Total Carbs: 62.9 g, Protein: 38.4 g.

111.Chicken Omelet

Servings: 2
Cooking Time: 16 Minutes
Ingredients:
- 1 teaspoon butter
- 1 small yellow onion, chopped
- ½ jalapeño pepper, seeded and chopped
- 3 eggs
- Salt and ground black pepper, as required
- ¼ cup cooked chicken, shredded

Directions:

1. In a frying pan, melt the butter over medium heat and cook the onion for about 4-5 minutes.
2. Add the jalapeño pepper and cook for about 1 minute.
3. Remove from the heat and set aside to cool slightly.
4. Meanwhile, in a bowl, add the eggs, salt, and black pepper and beat well.
5. Add the onion mixture and chicken and stir to combine.
6. Place the chicken mixture into a small baking pan.
7. Press "Power Button" of Air Fry Oven and turn the dial to select the "Air Fry" mode.
8. Press the Time button and again turn the dial to set the cooking time to 6 minutes.
9. Now push the Temp button and rotate the dial to set the temperature at 355 degrees F.
10. Press "Start/Pause" button to start.
11. When the unit beeps to show that it is preheated, open the lid.
12. Arrange pan over the "Wire Rack" and insert in the oven.
13. Cut the omelet into 2 portions and serve hot.
- **Nutrition Info:** Calories 153 Total Fat 9.1 g Saturated Fat 3.4 g Cholesterol 264 mg Sodium 196 mg Total Carbs 4 g Fiber 0.9 g Sugar 2.1 g Protein 13.8 g

112.Tomato-corn Frittata With Avocado Dressing

Servings:2 Or 3
Cooking Time: 20 Minutes
Ingredients:
- ½ cup cherry tomatoes, halved
- Kosher salt and freshly ground black pepper, to taste
- 6 large eggs, lightly beaten
- ½ cup fresh corn kernels
- ¼ cup milk
- 1 tablespoon finely chopped fresh dill
- ½ cup shredded Monterey Jack cheese
- Avocado Dressing:
- 1 ripe avocado, pitted and peeled
- 2 tablespoons fresh lime juice
- ¼ cup olive oil
- 1 scallion, finely chopped
- 8 fresh basil leaves, finely chopped

Directions:
1. Put the tomato halves in a colander and lightly season with salt. Set aside for 10 minutes to drain well. Pour the tomatoes into a large bowl and fold in the eggs, corn, milk, and dill. Sprinkle with salt and pepper and stir until mixed.
2. Pour the egg mixture into the baking pan.

3. Slide the baking pan into Rack Position 1, select Convection Bake, set temperature to 300ºF (150ºC) and set time to 15 minutes.
4. When done, remove the pan from the oven. Scatter the cheese on top.
5. Slide the baking pan into Rack Position 1, select Convection Bake, set temperature to 315ºF (157ºC) and set time to 5 minutes. Return the pan to the oven.
6. Meanwhile, make the avocado dressing: Mash the avocado with the lime juice in a medium bowl until smooth. Mix in the olive oil, scallion, and basil and stir until well incorporated.
7. When cooking is complete, the frittata will be puffy and set. Let the frittata cool for 5 minutes and serve alongside the avocado dressing.

113.Parmesan Asparagus

Servings:4
Cooking Time: 20 Minutes
Ingredients:
- 1 lb asparagus spears
- ¼ cup flour
- 1 cup breadcrumbs
- ½ cup Parmesan cheese, grated
- 2 eggs, beaten
- Salt and black pepper to taste

Directions:
1. Preheat on AirFry function to 370 F. Combine breadcrumbs, Parmesan cheese, salt, and pepper in a bowl. Line a baking sheet with parchment paper.
2. Dip the spears into the flour first, then into the eggs, and finally coat with the crumb mixture. Arrange them on a baking tray and press Start. Bake for 8-10 minutes. Serve warm.

114.Fried Churros With Cinnamon

Servings:x
Cooking Time:x
Ingredients:
- ¼ cup (55g) unsalted butter, melted
- ½ cup (100g) sugar
- ½ teaspoon ground cinnamon
- Special equipment
- Piping bag
- X-inch (1.5cm) closed star pastry tip
- 1 cup (240ml) water
- 1 tablespoon (15g) unsalted butter
- 1 tablespoon sugar
- ½ teaspoon vanilla extract
- ¼ teaspoon kosher salt
- 1 cup (130g) all-purpose flour
- 1 egg
- Scissors

Directions:

1. Combine water, butter, sugar, vanilla, and salt in large saucepan and bring to boil over medium-high heat. Add flour all at once and stir with wooden spoon until well combined, with no streaks of flour remaining. Transfer dough to bowl of stand mixer fitted with paddle attachment.

2. Mix on medium-high speed until cooled slightly, about 1 minute.

3. Reduce speed to low and add egg. Once egg is incorporated, increase speed to high and beat until outside of bowl is cool, about 12–15 minutes. Select AIRFRY/350°F (175°C)/SUPER CONVECTION/20 minutes and press START to preheat oven.

4. Transfer dough to piping bag fitted with X-inch (1.5cm) closed star pastry tip. Pipe 3-inch (7.5cm) lengths of dough onto air fry rack, using scissors to snip dough at tip. Cook in rack position 4 until churros are brown and crisp on the outside, about 20 minutes. Place melted butter in medium bowl. Combine sugar and cinnamon in a second medium bowl.

5. Toss warm churros in melted butter and then in cinnamon sugar. Pipe remaining dough onto air fry rack and repeat steps 5–7. Serve immediately with chocolate sauce or dulce de leche for dipping.

LUNCH RECIPES

115. Glazed Lamb Chops

Servings: 4
Cooking Time: 15 Minutes
Ingredients:
- 1 tablespoon Dijon mustard
- ½ tablespoon fresh lime juice
- 1 teaspoon honey
- ½ teaspoon olive oil
- Salt and ground black pepper, as required
- 4 (4-ounce) lamb loin chops

Directions:
1. In a black pepper large bowl, mix together the mustard, lemon juice, oil, honey, salt, and black pepper.
2. Add the chops and coat with the mixture generously.
3. Place the chops onto the greased "Sheet Pan".
4. Press "Power Button" of Ninja Foodi Digital Air Fry Oven and turn the dial to select the "Air Bake" mode.
5. Press the Time button and again turn the dial to set the cooking time to 15 minutes.
6. Now push the Temp button and rotate the dial to set the temperature at 390 degrees F.
7. Press "Start/Pause" button to start.
8. When the unit beeps to show that it is preheated, open the lid.
9. Insert the "Sheet Pan" in oven.
10. Flip the chops once halfway through.
11. Serve hot.
- **Nutrition Info:** Calories: 224 kcal Total Fat: 9.1 g Saturated Fat: 3.1 g Cholesterol: 102 mg Sodium: 169 mg Total Carbs: 1.7 g Fiber: 0.1 g Sugar: 1.5 g Protein: 32 g

116. Cheddar & Cream Omelet

Servings: 2
Cooking Time: 8 Minutes
Ingredients:
- 4 eggs
- ¼ cup cream
- Salt and ground black pepper, as required
- ¼ cup Cheddar cheese, grated

Directions:
1. In a bowl, add the eggs, cream, salt, and black pepper and beat well.
2. Place the egg mixture into a small baking pan.
3. Press "Power Button" of Air Fry Oven and turn the dial to select the "Air Fry" mode.
4. Press the Time button and again turn the dial to set the cooking time to 8 minutes.
5. Now push the Temp button and rotate the dial to set the temperature at 350 degrees F.
6. Press "Start/Pause" button to start.

7. When the unit beeps to show that it is preheated, open the lid.
8. Arrange pan over the "Wire Rack" and insert in the oven.
9. After 4 minutes, sprinkle the omelet with cheese evenly.
10. Cut the omelet into 2 portions and serve hot.
11. Cut into equal-sized wedges and serve hot.
- **Nutrition Info:** Calories: 202 Cal Total Fat: 15.1 g Saturated Fat: 6.8 g Cholesterol: 348 mg Sodium: 298 mg Total Carbs: 1.8 g Fiber: 0 g Sugar: 1.4 g Protein: 14.8 g

117. Cheese-stuffed Meatballs

Servings: 4
Cooking Time: 10 Minutes
Ingredients:
- ⅓ cup soft bread crumbs
- 3 tablespoons milk
- 1 tablespoon ketchup
- 1 egg
- ½ teaspoon dried marjoram
- Pinch salt
- Freshly ground black pepper
- 1-pound 95 percent lean ground beef
- 20 ½-inch cubes of cheese
- Olive oil for misting

Directions:
1. Preparing the ingredients. In a large bowl, combine the bread crumbs, milk, ketchup, egg, marjoram, salt, and pepper, and mix well. Add the ground beef and mix gently but thoroughly with your hands. Form the mixture into 20 meatballs. Shape each meatball around a cheese cube. Mist the meatballs with olive oil and put into the instant crisp air fryer basket.
2. Air frying. Close air fryer lid. Bake for 10 to 13 minutes or until the meatballs register 165°f on a meat thermometer.
- **Nutrition Info:** Calories: 393; Fat: 17g; Protein:50g; Fiber:0g

118. Herb-roasted Chicken Tenders

Servings: 2
Cooking Time: 10 Minutes
Ingredients:
- 7 ounces chicken tenders
- 1 tablespoon olive oil
- 1/2 teaspoon Herbes de Provence
- 2 tablespoons Dijon mustard
- 1 tablespoon honey
- Salt and pepper

Directions:
1. Start by preheating toaster oven to 450°F.
2. Brush bottom of pan with 1/2 tablespoon olive oil.

3. Season the chicken with herbs, salt, and pepper.
4. Place the chicken in a single flat layer in the pan and drizzle the remaining olive oil over it.
5. Bake for about 10 minutes.
6. While the chicken is baking, mix together the mustard and honey for a tasty condiment.

- **Nutrition Info:** Calories: 297, Sodium: 268 mg, Dietary Fiber: 0.8 g, Total Fat: 15.5 g, Total Carbs: 9.6 g, Protein: 29.8 g.

119.Turkey-stuffed Peppers

Servings: 6
Cooking Time: 35 Minutes
Ingredients:
- 1 pound lean ground turkey
- 1 tablespoon olive oil
- 2 cloves garlic, minced
- 1/3 onion, minced
- 1 tablespoon cilantro (optional)
- 1 teaspoon garlic powder
- 1 teaspoon cumin powder
- 1/2 teaspoon salt
- Pepper to taste
- 3 large red bell peppers
- 1 cup chicken broth
- 1/4 cup tomato sauce
- 1-1/2 cups cooked brown rice
- 1/4 cup shredded cheddar
- 6 green onions

Directions:
1. Start by preheating toaster oven to 400°F.
2. Heat a skillet on medium heat.
3. Add olive oil to the skillet, then mix in onion and garlic.
4. Sauté for about 5 minutes, or until the onion starts to look opaque.
5. Add the turkey to the skillet and season with cumin, garlic powder, salt, and pepper.
6. Brown the meat until thoroughly cooked, then mix in chicken broth and tomato sauce.
7. Reduce heat and simmer for about 5 minutes, stirring occasionally.
8. Add the brown rice and continue stirring until it is evenly spread through the mix.
9. Cut the bell peppers lengthwise down the middle and remove all of the seeds.
10. Grease a pan or line it with parchment paper and lay all peppers in the pan with the outside facing down.
11. Spoon the meat mixture evenly into each pepper and use the back of the spoon to level.
12. Bake for 30 minutes.
13. Remove pan from oven and sprinkle cheddar over each pepper, then put it back in for another 3 minutes, or until the cheese is melted.
14. While the cheese melts, dice the green onions. Remove pan from oven and sprinkle onions over each pepper and serve.

- **Nutrition Info:** Calories: 394, Sodium: 493 mg, Dietary Fiber: 4.1 g, Total Fat: 12.9 g, Total Carbs: 44.4 g, Protein: 27.7 g.

120.Chicken Legs With Dilled Brussels Sprouts

Servings: 2
Cooking Time: 10 Minutes
Ingredients:
- 2 chicken legs
- 1/2 teaspoon paprika
- 1/2 teaspoon kosher salt
- 1/2 teaspoon black pepper
- 1/2 pound Brussels sprouts
- 1 teaspoon dill, fresh or dried

Directions:
1. Start by preheating your Air Fryer to 370 degrees F.
2. Now, season your chicken with paprika, salt, and pepper. Transfer the chicken legs to the cooking basket. Cook for 10 minutes.
3. Flip the chicken legs and cook an additional 10 minutes. Reserve.
4. Add the Brussels sprouts to the cooking basket; sprinkle with dill. Cook at 380 degrees F for 15 minutes, shaking the basket halfway through.
5. Serve with the reserved chicken legs.

- **Nutrition Info:** 365 Calories; 21g Fat; 3g Carbs; 36g Protein; 2g Sugars; 3g Fiber

121.Air Fried Sausages

Servings: 6
Cooking Time: 13 Minutes
Ingredients:
- 6 sausage
- olive oil spray

Directions:
1. Pour 5 cup of water into Instant Pot Duo Crisp Air Fryer. Place air fryer basket inside the pot, spray inside with nonstick spray and put sausage links inside.
2. Close the Air Fryer lid and steam for about 5 minutes.
3. Remove the lid once done. Spray links with olive oil and close air crisp lid.
4. Set to air crisp at 400°F for 8 min flipping halfway through so both sides get browned.

- **Nutrition Info:** Calories 267, Total Fat 23g, Total Carbs 2g, Protein 13g

122.Pecan Crunch Catfish And Asparagus

Servings: 4
Cooking Time: 12 Minutes

Ingredients:
- 1 cup whole wheat panko breadcrumbs
- 1/4 cup chopped pecans
- 3 teaspoons chopped fresh thyme
- 1-1/2 tablespoons extra-virgin olive oil, plus more for the pan
- Salt and pepper to taste
- 1-1/4 pounds asparagus
- 1 tablespoon honey
- 4 (5- to 6-ounce each) catfish filets

Directions:
1. Start by preheating toaster oven to 425°F.
2. Combine breadcrumbs, pecans, 2 teaspoons thyme, 1 tablespoon oil, salt, pepper and 2 tablespoons water.
3. In another bowl combine asparagus, the rest of the thyme, honey, salt, and pepper.
4. Spread the asparagus in a flat layer on a baking sheet. Sprinkle a quarter of the breadcrumb mixture over the asparagus.
5. Lay the catfish over the asparagus and press the rest of the breadcrumb mixture into each piece. Roast for 12 minutes.
- **Nutrition Info:** Calories: 531, Sodium: 291 mg, Dietary Fiber: 6.1 g, Total Fat: 30.4 g, Total Carbs: 31.9 g, Protein: 34.8 g.

123.Herbed Radish Sauté(3)

Servings: 4
Cooking Time: 12 Minutes
Ingredients:
- 2 bunches red radishes; halved
- 2 tbsp. parsley; chopped.
- 2 tbsp. balsamic vinegar
- 1 tbsp. olive oil
- Salt and black pepper to taste.

Directions:
1. Take a bowl and mix the radishes with the remaining ingredients except the parsley, toss and put them in your air fryer's basket.
2. Cook at 400°F for 15 minutes, divide between plates, sprinkle the parsley on top and serve as a side dish
- **Nutrition Info:** Calories: 180; Fat: 4g; Fiber: 2g; Carbs: 3g; Protein: 5g

124.Turkey And Broccoli Stew

Servings: 4
Cooking Time: 12 Minutes
Ingredients:
- 1 broccoli head, florets separated
- 1 turkey breast, skinless; boneless and cubed
- 1 cup tomato sauce
- 1 tbsp. parsley; chopped.
- 1 tbsp. olive oil
- Salt and black pepper to taste.

Directions:

1. In a baking dish that fits your air fryer, mix the turkey with the rest of the ingredients except the parsley, toss, introduce the dish in the fryer, bake at 380°F for 25 minutes
2. Divide into bowls, sprinkle the parsley on top and serve.
- **Nutrition Info:** Calories: 250; Fat: 11g; Fiber: 2g; Carbs: 6g; Protein: 12g

125.Spice-roasted Almonds

Servings: 32
Cooking Time: 10 Minutes
Ingredients:
- 1 tablespoon chili powder
- 1 tablespoon olive oil
- 1/2 teaspoon salt
- 1/2 teaspoon ground cumin
- 1/2 teaspoon ground coriander
- 1/4 teaspoon ground cinnamon
- 1/4 teaspoon black pepper
- 2 cups whole almonds

Directions:
1. Start by preheating toaster oven to 350°F.
2. Mix olive oil, chili powder, coriander, cinnamon, cumin, salt, and pepper.
3. Add almonds and toss together.
4. Transfer to a baking pan and bake for 10 minutes.
- **Nutrition Info:** Calories: 39, Sodium: 37 mg, Dietary Fiber: 0.8 g, Total Fat: 3.5 g, Total Carbs: 1.4 g, Protein: 1.3 g.

126.Herb-roasted Turkey Breast

Servings: 8
Cooking Time: 60 Minutes
Ingredients:
- 3 lb turkey breast
- Rub Ingredients:
- 2 tbsp olive oil
- 2 tbsp lemon juice
- 1 tbsp minced Garlic
- 2 tsp ground mustard
- 2 tsp kosher salt
- 1 tsp pepper
- 1 tsp dried rosemary
- 1 tsp dried thyme
- 1 tsp ground sage

Directions:
1. Take a small bowl and thoroughly combine the Rub Ingredients: in it. Rub this on the outside of the turkey breast and under any loose skin.
2. Place the coated turkey breast keeping skin side up on a cooking tray.
3. Place the drip pan at the bottom of the cooking chamber of the Instant Pot Duo Crisp Air Fryer. Select Air Fry option, post this, adjust the temperature to 360°F and the time to one hour, then touch start.

4. When preheated, add the food to the cooking tray in the lowest position. Close the lid for cooking.
5. When the Air Fry program is complete, check to make sure that the thickest portion of the meat reads at least 160°F, remove the turkey and let it rest for 10 minutes before slicing and serving.
- **Nutrition Info:** Calories 214, Total Fat 10g, Total Carbs 2g, Protein 29g

127. Lobster Tails

Servings: 2
Cooking Time: 8 Minutes
Ingredients:
- 2 6oz lobster tails
- 1 tsp salt
- 1 tsp chopped chives
- 2 Tbsp unsalted butter melted
- 1 Tbsp minced garlic
- 1 tsp lemon juice

Directions:
1. Combine butter, garlic, salt, chives, and lemon juice to prepare butter mixture.
2. Butterfly lobster tails by cutting through shell followed by removing the meat and resting it on top of the shell.
3. Place them on the tray in the Instant Pot Duo Crisp Air Fryer basket and spread butter over the top of lobster meat. Close the Air Fryer lid, select the Air Fry option and cook on 380°F for 4 minutes.
4. Open the Air Fryer lid and spread more butter on top, cook for extra 2-4 minutes until done.
- **Nutrition Info:** Calories 120, Total Fat 12g, Total Carbs 2g, Protein 1g

128. Spicy Egg And Ground Turkey Bake

Servings: 6
Cooking Time: 10 Minutes
Ingredients:
- 1½ pounds ground turkey
- 6 whole eggs, well beaten
- 1/3 teaspoon smoked paprika
- 2 egg whites, beaten
- Tabasco sauce, for drizzling
- 2 tablespoons sesame oil
- 2 leeks, chopped
- 3 cloves garlic, finely minced
- 1 teaspoon ground black pepper
- 1/2 teaspoon sea salt

Directions:
1. Warm the oil in a pan over moderate heat; then, sweat the leeks and garlic until tender; stir periodically.
2. Next, grease 6 oven safe ramekins with pan spray. Divide the sautéed mixture among six ramekins.

3. In a bowl, beat the eggs and egg whites using a wire whisk. Stir in the smoked paprika, salt and black pepper; whisk until everything is thoroughly combined. Divide the egg mixture among the ramekins.
4. Air-fry approximately 22 minutes at 345 degrees F. Drizzle Tabasco sauce over each portion and serve.
- **Nutrition Info:** 298 Calories; 16g Fat; 4g Carbs; 16g Protein; 9g Sugars; 7g Fiber

129. Crisp Chicken Casserole

Servings: 4
Cooking Time: 15 Minutes
Ingredients:
- 3 cup chicken, shredded
- 12 oz bag egg noodles
- 1/2 large onion
- 1/2 cup chopped carrots
- 1/4 cup frozen peas
- 1/4 cup frozen broccoli pieces
- 2 stalks celery chopped
- 5 cup chicken broth
- 1 tsp garlic powder
- salt and pepper to taste
- 1 cup cheddar cheese, shredded
- 1 package French's onions
- 1/4 cup sour cream
- 1 can cream of chicken and mushroom soup

Directions:
1. Place the chicken, vegetables, garlic powder, salt and pepper, and broth and stir. Then place it into the Instant Pot Duo Crisp Air Fryer Basket.
2. Press or lightly stir the egg noodles into the mix until damp/wet.
3. Select the option Air Fryer and cook for 4 minutes.
4. Stir in the sour cream, can of soup, cheese, and 1/3 of the French's onions.
5. Top with the remaining French's onions and close the Air Fryer lid and cook for about 10 more minutes.
- **Nutrition Info:** Calories 301, Total Fat 17g, Total Carbs 17g, Protein 20g

130. Garlic Chicken Potatoes

Servings: 4
Cooking Time: 30 Minutes
Ingredients:
- 2 lbs. red potatoes, quartered
- 3 tablespoons olive oil
- 1/2 teaspoon cumin seeds
- Salt and black pepper, to taste
- 4 garlic cloves, chopped
- 2 tablespoons brown sugar
- 1 lemon (1/2 juiced and 1/2 cut into wedges)
- Pinch of red pepper flakes

- 4 skinless, boneless chicken breasts
- 2 tablespoons cilantro, chopped

Directions:
1. Place the chicken, lemon, garlic, and potatoes in a baking pan.
2. Toss the spices, herbs, oil, and sugar in a bowl.
3. Add this mixture to the chicken and veggies then toss well to coat.
4. Press "Power Button" of Air Fry Oven and turn the dial to select the "Bake" mode.
5. Press the Time button and again turn the dial to set the cooking time to 30 minutes.
6. Now push the Temp button and rotate the dial to set the temperature at 400 degrees F.
7. Once preheated, place the baking pan inside and close its lid.
8. Serve warm.
- **Nutrition Info:** Calories 545 Total Fat 36.4 g Saturated Fat 10.1 g Cholesterol 200 mg Sodium 272 mg Total Carbs 40.7 g Fiber 0.2 g Sugar 0.1 g Protein 42.5 g

131. Parmigiano Reggiano And Prosciutto Toasts With Balsamic Glaze

Servings: 8
Cooking Time: 15 Minutes
Ingredients:
- 3 ounces thinly sliced prosciutto, cut crosswise into 1/4-inch-wide strips
- 1 (3-ounce) piece Parmigiano Reggiano cheese
- 1/2 cup balsamic vinegar
- 1 medium red onion, thinly sliced
- 1 loaf ciabatta, cut into 3/4-inch-thick slices
- 1 tablespoon extra-virgin olive oil
- 1 clove garlic
- Black pepper to taste

Directions:
1. Preheat toaster oven to 350°F.
2. Place onion in a bowl of cold water and let sit for 10 minutes.
3. Bring vinegar to a boil, then reduce heat and simmer for 5 minutes.
4. Remove from heat completely and set aside to allow the vinegar to thicken.
5. Drain the onion.
6. Brush the tops of each bun with oil, rub with garlic, and sprinkle with pepper.
7. Use a vegetable peeler to make large curls of Parmigiano Reggiano cheese and place them on the bun.
8. Bake for 15 minutes or until the bread just starts to crisp.
9. Sprinkle prosciutto and onions on top, then drizzle vinegar and serve.
- **Nutrition Info:** Calories: 154, Sodium: 432 mg, Dietary Fiber: 1.0 g, Total Fat: 5.6 g, Total Carbs: 17.3 g, Protein: 8.1 g.

132. Creamy Green Beans And Tomatoes

Servings: 4
Cooking Time: 20 Minutes
Ingredients:
- 1 pound green beans, trimmed and halved
- ½ pound cherry tomatoes, halved
- 2 tablespoons olive oil
- 1 teaspoon oregano, dried
- 1 teaspoon basil, dried
- Salt and black pepper to the taste
- 1 cup heavy cream
- ½ tablespoon cilantro, chopped

Directions:
1. In your air fryer's pan, combine the green beans with the tomatoes and the other Ingredients:, toss and cook at 360 degrees F for 20 minutes.
2. Divide the mix between plates and serve.
- **Nutrition Info:** Calories 174, fat 5, fiber 7, carbs 11, protein 4

133. Turkey Meatballs With Manchego Cheese

Servings: 4
Cooking Time: 10 Minutes
Ingredients:
- 1 pound ground turkey
- 1/2 pound ground pork
- 1 egg, well beaten
- 1 teaspoon dried basil
- 1 teaspoon dried rosemary
- 1/4 cup Manchego cheese, grated
- 2 tablespoons yellow onions, finely chopped
- 1 teaspoon fresh garlic, finely chopped
- Sea salt and ground black pepper, to taste

Directions:
1. In a mixing bowl, combine all the ingredients until everything is well incorporated.
2. Shape the mixture into 1-inch balls.
3. Cook the meatballs in the preheated Air Fryer at 380 degrees for 7 minutes. Shake halfway through the cooking time. Work in batches.
4. Serve with your favorite pasta.
- **Nutrition Info:** 386 Calories; 24g Fat; 9g Carbs; 41g Protein; 3g Sugars; 2g Fiber

134. Turkey Meatloaf

Servings: 4
Cooking Time: 20 Minutes
Ingredients:
- 1 pound ground turkey
- 1 cup kale leaves, trimmed and finely chopped
- 1 cup onion, chopped
- ½ cup fresh breadcrumbs
- 1 cup Monterey Jack cheese, grated

- 2 garlic cloves, minced
- ¼ cup salsa verde
- 1 teaspoon red chili powder
- ½ teaspoon ground cumin
- ½ teaspoon dried oregano, crushed
- Salt and ground black pepper, as required

Directions:
1. Preheat the Air fryer to 400 degree F and grease an Air fryer basket.
2. Mix all the ingredients in a bowl and divide the turkey mixture into 4 equal-sized portions.
3. Shape each into a mini loaf and arrange the loaves into the Air fryer basket.
4. Cook for about 20 minutes and dish out to serve warm.
- **Nutrition Info:** Calories: 435, Fat: 23.1g, Carbohydrates: 18.1g, Sugar: 3.6g, Protein: 42.2g, Sodium: 641mg

135.Skinny Black Bean Flautas

Servings: 10
Cooking Time: 25 Minutes
Ingredients:
- 2 (15-ounce) cans black beans
- 1 cup shredded cheddar
- 1 (4-ounce) can diced green chilies
- 2 teaspoons taco seasoning
- 10 (8-inch) whole wheat flour tortillas
- Olive oil

Directions:
1. Start by preheating toaster oven to 350°F.
2. Drain black beans and mash in a medium bowl with a fork.
3. Mix in cheese, chilies, and taco seasoning until all ingredients are thoroughly combined.
4. Evenly spread the mixture over each tortilla and wrap tightly.
5. Brush each side lightly with olive oil and place on a baking sheet.
6. Bake for 12 minutes, turn, and bake for another 13 minutes.
- **Nutrition Info:** Calories: 367, Sodium: 136 mg, Dietary Fiber: 14.4 g, Total Fat: 2.8 g, Total Carbs: 64.8 g, Protein: 22.6 g.

136.Air Fryer Marinated Salmon

Servings: 4
Cooking Time: 12 Minutes
Ingredients:
- 4 salmon fillets or 1 1lb fillet cut into 4 pieces
- 1 Tbsp brown sugar
- ½ Tbsp Minced Garlic
- 6 Tbsps Soy Sauce
- ¼ cup Dijon Mustard
- 1 Green onions finely chopped

Directions:

1. Take a bowl and whisk together soy sauce, dijon mustard, brown sugar, and minced garlic. Pour this mixture over salmon fillets, making sure that all the fillets are covered. Refrigerate and marinate for 20-30 minutes.
2. Remove salmon fillets from marinade and place them in greased or lined on the tray in the Instant Pot Duo Crisp Air Fryer basket, close the lid.
3. Select the Air Fry option and Air Fry for around 12 minutes at 400°F.
4. Remove from Instant Pot Duo Crisp Air Fryer and top with chopped green onions.
- **Nutrition Info:** Calories 267, Total Fat 11g, Total Carbs 5g, Protein 37g

137.Boneless Air Fryer Turkey Breasts

Servings: 4
Cooking Time: 50 Minutes
Ingredients:
- 3 lb boneless breast
- ¼ cup mayonnaise
- 2 tsp poultry seasoning
- 1 tsp salt
- ½ tsp garlic powder
- ¼ tsp black pepper

Directions:
1. Choose the Air Fry option on the Instant Pot Duo Crisp Air fryer. Set the temperature to 360°F and push start. The preheating will start.
2. Season your boneless turkey breast with mayonnaise, poultry seasoning, salt, garlic powder, and black pepper.
3. Once preheated, Air Fry the turkey breasts on 360°F for 1 hour, turning every 15 minutes or until internal temperature has reached a temperature of 165°F.
- **Nutrition Info:** Calories 558, Total Fat 18g, Total Carbs 1g, Protein 98g

138.Roasted Garlic(2)

Servings: 12 Cloves
Cooking Time: 12 Minutes
Ingredients:
- 1 medium head garlic
- 2 tsp. avocado oil

Directions:
1. Remove any hanging excess peel from the garlic but leave the cloves covered. Cut off ¼ of the head of garlic, exposing the tips of the cloves
2. Drizzle with avocado oil. Place the garlic head into a small sheet of aluminum foil, completely enclosing it. Place it into the air fryer basket. Adjust the temperature to 400 Degrees F and set the timer for 20 minutes. If your garlic head is a bit smaller, check it after 15 minutes

3. When done, garlic should be golden brown and very soft
4. To serve, cloves should pop out and easily be spread or sliced. Store in an airtight container in the refrigerator up to 5 days.
5. You may also freeze individual cloves on a baking sheet, then store together in a freezer-safe storage bag once frozen.
- **Nutrition Info:** Calories: 11; Protein: 2g; Fiber: 1g; Fat: 7g; Carbs: 0g

139.Orange Chicken Rice

Servings: 4
Cooking Time: 55 Minutes
Ingredients:
- 3 tablespoons olive oil
- 1 medium onion, chopped
- 1 3/4 cups chicken broth
- 1 cup brown basmati rice
- Zest and juice of 2 oranges
- Salt to taste
- 4 (6-oz.) boneless, skinless chicken thighs
- Black pepper, to taste
- 2 tablespoons fresh mint, chopped
- 2 tablespoons pine nuts, toasted

Directions:
1. Spread the rice in a casserole dish and place the chicken on top.
2. Toss the rest of the Ingredients: in a bowl and liberally pour over the chicken.
3. Press "Power Button" of Air Fry Oven and turn the dial to select the "Bake" mode.
4. Press the Time button and again turn the dial to set the cooking time to 55 minutes.
5. Now push the Temp button and rotate the dial to set the temperature at 350 degrees F.
6. Once preheated, place the casserole dish inside and close its lid.
7. Serve warm.
- **Nutrition Info:** Calories 231 Total Fat 20.1 g Saturated Fat 2.4 g Cholesterol 110 mg Sodium 941 mg Total Carbs 30.1 g Fiber 0.9 g Sugar 1.4 g Protein 14.6 g

140.Rolled Salmon Sandwich

Servings: 1
Cooking Time: 5 Minutes
Ingredients:
- 1 piece of flatbread
- 1 salmon filet
- Pinch of salt
- 1 tablespoon green onion, chopped
- 1/4 teaspoon dried sumac
- 1/2 teaspoon thyme
- 1/2 teaspoon sesame seeds
- 1/4 English cucumber
- 1 tablespoon yogurt

Directions:

1. Start by peeling and chopping the cucumber. Cut the salmon at a 45-degree angle into 4 slices and lay them flat on the flatbread.
2. Sprinkle salmon with salt to taste. Sprinkle onions, thyme, sumac, and sesame seeds evenly over the salmon.
3. Broil the salmon for at least 3 minutes, but longer if you want a more well-done fish.
4. While you broil your salmon, mix together the yogurt and cucumber. Remove your flatbread from the toaster oven and put it on a plate, then spoon the yogurt mix over the salmon.
5. Fold the sides of the flatbread in and roll it up for a gourmet lunch that you can take on the go.
- **Nutrition Info:** Calories: 347, Sodium: 397 mg, Dietary Fiber: 1.6 g, Total Fat: 12.4 g, Total Carbs: 20.6 g, Protein: 38.9 g.

141.Green Bean Casserole(2)

Servings: 4
Cooking Time: 12 Minutes
Ingredients:
- 1 lb. fresh green beans, edges trimmed
- ½ oz. pork rinds, finely ground
- 1 oz. full-fat cream cheese
- ½ cup heavy whipping cream.
- ¼ cup diced yellow onion
- ½ cup chopped white mushrooms
- ½ cup chicken broth
- 4 tbsp. unsalted butter.
- ¼ tsp. xanthan gum

Directions:
1. In a medium skillet over medium heat, melt the butter. Sauté the onion and mushrooms until they become soft and fragrant, about 3–5 minutes.
2. Add the heavy whipping cream, cream cheese and broth to the pan. Whisk until smooth. Bring to a boil and then reduce to a simmer. Sprinkle the xanthan gum into the pan and remove from heat
3. Chop the green beans into 2-inch pieces and place into a 4-cup round baking dish. Pour the sauce mixture over them and stir until coated. Top the dish with ground pork rinds. Place into the air fryer basket
4. Adjust the temperature to 320 Degrees F and set the timer for 15 minutes. Top will be golden and green beans fork tender when fully cooked. Serve warm.
- **Nutrition Info:** Calories: 267; Protein: 6g; Fiber: 2g; Fat: 24g; Carbs: 7g

142.Simple Turkey Breast

Servings: 10
Cooking Time: 40 Minutes
Ingredients:

- 1: 8-poundsbone-in turkey breast
- Salt and black pepper, as required
- 2 tablespoons olive oil

Directions:
1. Preheat the Air fryer to 360 degree F and grease an Air fryer basket.
2. Season the turkey breast with salt and black pepper and drizzle with oil.
3. Arrange the turkey breast into the Air Fryer basket, skin side down and cook for about 20 minutes.
4. Flip the side and cook for another 20 minutes.
5. Dish out in a platter and cut into desired size slices to serve.
- **Nutrition Info:** Calories: 719, Fat: 35.9g, Carbohydrates: 0g, Sugar: 0g, Protein: 97.2g, Sodium: 386mg

143.Pumpkin Pancakes

Servings: 4
Cooking Time: 12 Minutes
Ingredients:
- 1 square puff pastry
- 3 tablespoons pumpkin filling
- 1 small egg, beaten

Directions:
1. Roll out a square of puff pastry and layer it with pumpkin pie filling, leaving about ¼-inch space around the edges.
2. Cut it up into 8 equal sized square pieces and coat the edges with beaten egg.
3. Press "Power Button" of Air Fry Oven and turn the dial to select the "Air Fry" mode.
4. Press the Time button and again turn the dial to set the cooking time to 12 minutes.
5. Now push the Temp button and rotate the dial to set the temperature at 355 degrees F.
6. Press "Start/Pause" button to start.
7. When the unit beeps to show that it is preheated, open the lid.
8. Arrange the squares into a greased "Sheet Pan" and insert in the oven.
9. Serve warm.
- **Nutrition Info:** Calories: 109 Cal Total Fat: 6.7 g Saturated Fat: 1.8 g Cholesterol: 34 mg Sodium: 87 mg Total Carbs: 9.8 g Fiber: 0.5 g Sugar: 2.6 g Protein: 2.4 g

144.Pork Stew

Servings: 4
Cooking Time: 12 Minutes
Ingredients:
- 2 lb. pork stew meat; cubed
- 1 eggplant; cubed
- ½ cup beef stock
- 2 zucchinis; cubed
- ½ tsp. smoked paprika
- Salt and black pepper to taste.

- A handful cilantro; chopped.

Directions:
1. In a pan that fits your air fryer, mix all the ingredients, toss, introduce in your air fryer and cook at 370°F for 30 minutes
2. Divide into bowls and serve right away.
- **Nutrition Info:** Calories: 245; Fat: 12g; Fiber: 2g; Carbs: 5g; Protein: 14g

145.Coriander Artichokes(3)

Servings: 4
Cooking Time: 12 Minutes
Ingredients:
- 12 oz. artichoke hearts
- 1 tbsp. lemon juice
- 1 tsp. coriander, ground
- ½ tsp. cumin seeds
- ½ tsp. olive oil
- Salt and black pepper to taste.

Directions:
1. In a pan that fits your air fryer, mix all the ingredients, toss, introduce the pan in the fryer and cook at 370°F for 15 minutes
2. Divide the mix between plates and serve as a side dish.
- **Nutrition Info:** Calories: 200; Fat: 7g; Fiber: 2g; Carbs: 5g; Protein: 8g

146.Maple Chicken Thighs

Servings: 4
Cooking Time: 30 Minutes
Ingredients:
- 4 large chicken thighs, bone-in
- 2 tablespoons French mustard
- 2 tablespoons Dijon mustard
- 1 clove minced garlic
- 1/2 teaspoon dried marjoram
- 2 tablespoons maple syrup

Directions:
1. Mix chicken with everything in a bowl and coat it well.
2. Place the chicken along with its marinade in the baking pan.
3. Press "Power Button" of Air Fry Oven and turn the dial to select the "Bake" mode.
4. Press the Time button and again turn the dial to set the cooking time to 30 minutes.
5. Now push the Temp button and rotate the dial to set the temperature at 370 degrees F.
6. Once preheated, place the baking pan inside and close its lid.
7. Serve warm.
- **Nutrition Info:** Calories 301 Total Fat 15.8 g Saturated Fat 2.7 g Cholesterol 75 mg Sodium 189 mg Total Carbs 31.7 g Fiber 0.3 g Sugar 0.1 g Protein 28.2 g

147.Beer Coated Duck Breast

Servings: 2

Cooking Time: 20 Minutes

Ingredients:
- 1 tablespoon fresh thyme, chopped
- 1 cup beer
- 1: 10½-ouncesduck breast
- 6 cherry tomatoes
- 1 tablespoon olive oil
- 1 teaspoon mustard
- Salt and ground black pepper, as required
- 1 tablespoon balsamic vinegar

Directions:
1. Preheat the Air fryer to 390 degree F and grease an Air fryer basket.
2. Mix the olive oil, mustard, thyme, beer, salt, and black pepper in a bowl.
3. Coat the duck breasts generously with marinade and refrigerate, covered for about 4 hours.
4. Cover the duck breasts and arrange into the Air fryer basket.
5. Cook for about 15 minutes and remove the foil from breast.
6. Set the Air fryer to 355 degree F and place the duck breast and tomatoes into the Air Fryer basket.
7. Cook for about 5 minutes and dish out the duck breasts and cherry tomatoes.
8. Drizzle with vinegar and serve immediately.
- **Nutrition Info:** Calories: 332, Fat: 13.7g, Carbohydrates: 9.2g, Sugar: 2.5g, Protein: 34.6g, Sodium: 88mg

148.Okra And Green Beans Stew

Servings: 4
Cooking Time: 12 Minutes

Ingredients:
- 1 lb. green beans; halved
- 4 garlic cloves; minced
- 1 cup okra
- 3 tbsp. tomato sauce
- 1 tbsp. thyme; chopped.
- Salt and black pepper to taste.

Directions:
1. In a pan that fits your air fryer, mix all the ingredients, toss, introduce the pan in the air fryer and cook at 370°F for 15 minutes
2. Divide the stew into bowls and serve.
- **Nutrition Info:** Calories: 183; Fat: 5g; Fiber: 2g; Carbs: 4g; Protein: 8g

149.Basic Roasted Tofu

Servings: 4
Cooking Time: 45 Minutes

Ingredients:
- 1 or more (16-ounce) containers extra-firm tofu
- 1 tablespoon sesame oil
- 1 tablespoon soy sauce
- 1 tablespoon rice vinegar

- 1 tablespoon water

Directions:
1. Start by drying the tofu: first pat dry with paper towels, then lay on another set of paper towels or a dish towel.
2. Put a plate on top of the tofu then put something heavy on the plate (like a large can of vegetables). Leave it there for at least 20 minutes.
3. While tofu is being pressed, whip up marinade by combining oil, soy sauce, vinegar, and water in a bowl and set aside.
4. Cut the tofu into squares or sticks. Place the tofu in the marinade for at least 30 minutes.
5. Preheat toaster oven to 350°F. Line a pan with parchment paper and add as many pieces of tofu as you can, giving each piece adequate space.
6. Bake 20–45 minutes; tofu is done when the outside edges look golden brown. Time will vary depending on tofu size and shape.
- **Nutrition Info:** Calories: 114, Sodium: 239 mg, Dietary Fiber: 1.1 g, Total Fat: 8.1 g, Total Carbs: 2.2 g, Protein: 9.5 g.

150.Barbecue Air Fried Chicken

Servings: 10
Cooking Time: 26 Minutes

Ingredients:
- 1 teaspoon Liquid Smoke
- 2 cloves Fresh Garlic smashed
- 1/2 cup Apple Cider Vinegar
- 3 pounds Chuck Roast well-marbled with intramuscular fat
- 1 Tablespoon Kosher Salt
- 1 Tablespoon Freshly Ground Black Pepper
- 2 teaspoons Garlic Powder
- 1.5 cups Barbecue Sauce
- 1/4 cup Light Brown Sugar + more for sprinkling
- 2 Tablespoons Honey optional and in place of 2 TBL sugar

Directions:
1. Add meat to the Instant Pot Duo Crisp Air Fryer Basket, spreading out the meat.
2. Select the option Air Fry.
3. Close the Air Fryer lid and cook at 300 degrees F for 8 minutes. Pause the Air Fryer and flip meat over after 4 minutes.
4. Remove the lid and baste with more barbecue sauce and sprinkle with a little brown sugar.
5. Again Close the Air Fryer lid and set the temperature at 400°F for 9 minutes. Watch meat though the lid and flip it over after 5 minutes.
- **Nutrition Info:** Calories 360, Total Fat 16g, Total Carbs 27g, Protein 27g

151.Portobello Pesto Burgers

Servings: 4
Cooking Time: 26 Minutes
Ingredients:
- 4 portobello mushrooms
- 1/4 cup sundried tomato pesto
- 4 whole-grain hamburger buns
- 1 large ripe tomato
- 1 log fresh goat cheese
- 8 large fresh basil leaves

Directions:
1. Start by preheating toaster oven to 425°F.
2. Place mushrooms on a pan, round sides facing up.
3. Bake for 14 minutes.
4. Pull out tray, flip the mushrooms and spread 1 tablespoon of pesto on each piece.
5. Return to oven and bake for another 10 minutes.
6. Remove the mushrooms and toast the buns for 2 minutes.
7. Remove the buns and build the burger by placing tomatoes, mushroom, 2 slices of cheese, and a sprinkle of basil, then topping with the top bun.
- **Nutrition Info:** Calories: 297, Sodium: 346 mg, Dietary Fiber: 1.8 g, Total Fat: 18.1 g, Total Carbs: 19.7 g, Protein: 14.4 g.

152.Chili Chicken Sliders

Servings: 4
Cooking Time: 10 Minutes
Ingredients:
- 1/3 teaspoon paprika
- 1/3 cup scallions, peeled and chopped
- 3 cloves garlic, peeled and minced
- 1 teaspoon ground black pepper, or to taste
- 1/2 teaspoon fresh basil, minced
- 1 ½ cups chicken,minced
- 1 ½ tablespoons coconut aminos
- 1/2 teaspoon grated fresh ginger
- 1/2 tablespoon chili sauce
- 1 teaspoon salt

Directions:
1. Thoroughly combine all ingredients in a mixing dish. Then, form into 4 patties.
2. Cook in the preheated Air Fryer for 18 minutes at 355 degrees F.
3. Garnish with toppings of choice.
- **Nutrition Info:** 366 Calories; 6g Fat; 4g Carbs; 66g Protein; 3g Sugars; 9g Fiber

153.Spanish Chicken Bake

Servings: 4
Cooking Time: 25 Minutes
Ingredients:
- ½ onion, quartered
- ½ red onion, quartered
- ½ lb. potatoes, quartered
- 4 garlic cloves
- 4 tomatoes, quartered
- 1/8 cup chorizo
- ¼ teaspoon paprika powder
- 4 chicken thighs, boneless
- ¼ teaspoon dried oregano
- ½ green bell pepper, julienned
- Salt
- Black pepper

Directions:
1. Toss chicken, veggies, and all the Ingredients: in a baking tray.
2. Press "Power Button" of Air Fry Oven and turn the dial to select the "Bake" mode.
3. Press the Time button and again turn the dial to set the cooking time to 25 minutes.
4. Now push the Temp button and rotate the dial to set the temperature at 425 degrees F.
5. Once preheated, place the baking pan inside and close its lid.
6. Serve warm.
- **Nutrition Info:** Calories 301 Total Fat 8.9 g Saturated Fat 4.5 g Cholesterol 57 mg Sodium 340 mg Total Carbs 24.7 g Fiber 1.2 g Sugar 1.3 g Protein 15.3 g

154.Lemon Pepper Turkey

Servings: 6
Cooking Time: 45 Minutes
Ingredients:
- 3 lbs. turkey breast
- 2 tablespoons oil
- 1 tablespoon Worcestershire sauce
- 1 teaspoon lemon pepper
- 1/2 teaspoon salt

Directions:
1. Whisk everything in a bowl and coat the turkey liberally.
2. Place the turkey in the Air fryer basket.
3. Press "Power Button" of Air Fry Oven and turn the dial to select the "Air Fry" mode.
4. Press the Time button and again turn the dial to set the cooking time to 45 minutes.
5. Now push the Temp button and rotate the dial to set the temperature at 375 degrees F.
6. Once preheated, place the air fryer basket inside and close its lid.
7. Serve warm.
- **Nutrition Info:** Calories 391 Total Fat 2.8 g Saturated Fat 0.6 g Cholesterol 330 mg Sodium 62 mg Total Carbs 36.5 g Fiber 9.2 g Sugar 4.5 g Protein 6.6

155.Chicken & Rice Casserole

Servings: 6
Cooking Time: 40 Minutes
Ingredients:
- 2 lbs. bone-in chicken thighs
- Salt and black pepper

- 1 teaspoon olive oil
- 5 cloves garlic, chopped
- 2 large onions, chopped
- 2 large red bell peppers, chopped
- 1 tablespoon sweet Hungarian paprika
- 1 teaspoon hot Hungarian paprika
- 2 tablespoons tomato paste
- 2 cups chicken broth
- 3 cups brown rice, thawed
- 2 tablespoons parsley, chopped
- 6 tablespoons sour cream

Directions:
1. Mix broth, tomato paste, and all the spices in a bowl.
2. Add chicken and mix well to coat.
3. Spread the rice in a casserole dish and add chicken along with its marinade.
4. Top the casserole with the rest of the Ingredients:.
5. Press "Power Button" of Air Fry Oven and turn the dial to select the "Bake" mode.
6. Press the Time button and again turn the dial to set the cooking time to 40 minutes.
7. Now push the Temp button and rotate the dial to set the temperature at 350 degrees F.
8. Once preheated, place the baking pan inside and close its lid.
9. Serve warm.
- **Nutrition Info:** Calories 440 Total Fat 7.9 g Saturated Fat 1.8 g Cholesterol 5 mg Sodium 581 mg Total Carbs 21.8 g Sugar 7.1 g Fiber 2.6 g Protein 37.2 g

156.Roasted Delicata Squash With Kale

Servings: 2
Cooking Time: 10 Minutes
Ingredients:
- 1 medium delicata squash
- 1 bunch kale
- 1 clove garlic
- 2 tablespoons olive oil
- Salt and pepper

Directions:
1. Start by preheating toaster oven to 425°F.
2. Clean squash and cut off each end. Cut in half and remove the seeds. Quarter the halves.
3. Toss the squash in 1 tablespoon of olive oil.
4. Place the squash on a greased baking sheet and roast for 25 minutes, turning halfway through.
5. Rinse kale and remove stems. Chop garlic.
6. Heat the leftover oil in a medium skillet and add kale and salt to taste.
7. Sauté the kale until it darkens, then mix in the garlic.
8. Cook for another minute then remove from heat and add 2 tablespoons of water.

9. Remove squash from oven and lay it on top of the garlic kale.
10. Top with salt and pepper to taste and serve.
- **Nutrition Info:** Calories: 159, Sodium: 28 mg, Dietary Fiber: 1.8 g, Total Fat: 14.2 g, Total Carbs: 8.2 g, Protein: 2.6 g.

157.Fried Paprika Tofu

Servings:
Cooking Time: 12 Minutes
Ingredients:
- 1 block extra firm tofu; pressed to remove excess water and cut into cubes
- 1/4 cup cornstarch
- 1 tablespoon smoked paprika
- salt and pepper to taste

Directions:
1. Line the Air Fryer basket with aluminum foil and brush with oil. Preheat the Air Fryer to 370 - degrees Fahrenheit.
2. Mix all ingredients in a bowl. Toss to combine. Place in the Air Fryer basket and cook for 12 minutes.

158.Saucy Chicken With Leeks

Servings: 6
Cooking Time: 10 Minutes
Ingredients:
- 2 leeks, sliced
- 2 large-sized tomatoes, chopped
- 3 cloves garlic, minced
- ½ teaspoon dried oregano
- 6 chicken legs, boneless and skinless
- ½ teaspoon smoked cayenne pepper
- 2 tablespoons olive oil
- A freshly ground nutmeg

Directions:
1. In a mixing dish, thoroughly combine all ingredients, minus the leeks. Place in the refrigerator and let it marinate overnight.
2. Lay the leeks onto the bottom of an Air Fryer cooking basket. Top with the chicken legs.
3. Roast chicken legs at 375 degrees F for 18 minutes, turning halfway through. Serve with hoisin sauce.
- **Nutrition Info:** 390 Calories; 16g Fat; 2g Carbs; 59g Protein; 8g Sugars; 4g Fiber

159.Buttered Duck Breasts

Servings: 4
Cooking Time: 22 Minutes
Ingredients:
- 2: 12-ouncesduck breasts
- 3 tablespoons unsalted butter, melted
- Salt and ground black pepper, as required
- ½ teaspoon dried thyme, crushed
- ¼ teaspoon star anise powder

Directions:

1. Preheat the Air fryer to 390 degree F and grease an Air fryer basket.
2. Season the duck breasts generously with salt and black pepper.
3. Arrange the duck breasts into the prepared Air fryer basket and cook for about 10 minutes.
4. Dish out the duck breasts and drizzle with melted butter.
5. Season with thyme and star anise powder and place the duck breasts again into the Air fryer basket.
6. Cook for about 12 more minutes and dish out to serve warm.
- **Nutrition Info:** Calories: 296, Fat: 15.5g, Carbohydrates: 0.1g, Sugar: 0g, Protein: 37.5g, Sodium: 100mg

160.Buttery Artichokes

Servings: 4
Cooking Time: 20 Minutes
Ingredients:
- 4 artichokes, trimmed and halved
- 3 garlic cloves, minced
- 1 tablespoon olive oil
- Salt and black pepper to the taste
- 4 tablespoons butter, melted
- ¼ teaspoon cumin, ground
- 1 tablespoon lemon zest, grated

Directions:
1. In a bowl, combine the artichokes with the oil, garlic and the other Ingredients:, toss well and transfer them to the air fryer's basket.
2. Cook for 20 minutes at 370 degrees F, divide between plates and serve as a side dish.
- **Nutrition Info:** Calories 214, fat 5, fiber 8, carbs 12, protein 5

161.Simple Lamb Bbq With Herbed Salt

Servings: 8
Cooking Time: 1 Hour 20 Minutes
Ingredients:
- 2 ½ tablespoons herb salt
- 2 tablespoons olive oil
- 4 pounds boneless leg of lamb, cut into 2-inch chunks

Directions:
1. Preheat the air fryer to 390 ºF.
2. Place the grill pan accessory in the air fryer.
3. Season the meat with the herb salt and brush with olive oil.
4. Grill the meat for 20 minutes per batch.
5. Make sure to flip the meat every 10 minutes for even cooking.
- **Nutrition Info:** Calories: 347 kcal Total Fat: 17.8 g Saturated Fat: 0 g Cholesterol: 0 mg

Sodium: 0 mg Total Carbs: 0 g Fiber: 0 g Sugar: 0 g Protein: 46.6 g

162.Philly Cheesesteak Egg Rolls

Servings: 4-5
Cooking Time: 20 Minutes
Ingredients:
- 1 egg
- 1 tablespoon milk
- 2 tablespoons olive oil
- 1 small red onion
- 1 small red bell pepper
- 1 small green bell pepper
- 1 pound thinly slice roast beef
- 8 ounces shredded pepper jack cheese
- 8 ounces shredded provolone cheese
- 8-10 egg roll skins
- Salt and pepper

Directions:
1. Start by preheating toaster oven to 425°F.
2. Mix together egg and milk in a shallow bowl and set aside for later use.
3. Chop onions and bell peppers into small pieces.
4. Heat the oil in a medium sauce pan and add the onions and peppers.
5. Cook onions and peppers for 2–3 minutes until softened.
6. Add roast beef to the pan and sauté for another 5 minutes.
7. Add salt and pepper to taste.
8. Add cheese and mix together until melted.
9. Remove from heat and drain liquid from pan.
10. Roll the egg roll skins flat.
11. Add equal parts of the mix to each egg roll and roll them up per the instructions on the package.
12. Brush each egg roll with the egg mixture.
13. Line a pan with parchment paper and lay egg rolls seam-side down with a gap between each roll.
14. Bake for 20–25 minutes, depending on your preference of egg roll crispness.
- **Nutrition Info:** Calories: 769, Sodium: 1114 mg, Dietary Fiber: 2.1 g, Total Fat: 39.9 g, Total Carbs: 41.4 g, Protein: 58.4 g.

163.Bok Choy And Butter Sauce(1)

Servings: 4
Cooking Time: 12 Minutes
Ingredients:
- 2 bok choy heads; trimmed and cut into strips
- 1 tbsp. butter; melted
- 2 tbsp. chicken stock
- 1 tsp. lemon juice
- 1 tbsp. olive oil
- A pinch of salt and black pepper

Directions:
1. In a pan that fits your air fryer, mix all the ingredients, toss, introduce the pan in the air fryer and cook at 380°F for 15 minutes.
2. Divide between plates and serve as a side dish
- **Nutrition Info:** Calories: 141; Fat: 3g; Fiber: 2g; Carbs: 4g; Protein: 3g

164.Roasted Fennel, Ditalini, And Shrimp

Servings: 4
Cooking Time: 30 Minutes
Ingredients:
- 1 pound extra large, thawed, tail-on shrimp
- 1 teaspoon fennel seeds
- 1 teaspoon salt
- 1 fennel bulb, halved and sliced crosswise
- 4 garlic cloves, chopped
- 2 tablespoons olive oil
- 1/2 teaspoon freshly ground black pepper
- Grated zest of 1 lemon
- 1/2 pound whole wheat ditalini

Directions:
1. Start by preheating toaster oven to 450°F.
2. Toast the seeds in a medium pan over medium heat for about 5 minutes, then toss with shrimp.
3. Add water and 1/2 teaspoon salt to the pan and bring the mixture to a boil.
4. Reduce heat and simmer for 30 minutes.
5. Combine fennel, garlic, oil, pepper, and remaining salt in a roasting pan.
6. Roast for 20 minutes, then add shrimp mixture and roast for another 5 minutes or until shrimp are cooked.
7. While the fennel is roasting, cook pasta per the directions on the package, drain, and set aside.
8. Remove the shrimp mixture and mix in pasta, roast for another 5 minutes.
- **Nutrition Info:** Calories: 420, Sodium: 890 mg, Dietary Fiber: 4.2 g, Total Fat: 10.2 g, Total Carbs: 49.5 g, Protein: 33.9 g.

165.Sweet & Sour Pork

Servings: 4
Cooking Time: 27 Minutes
Ingredients:
- 2 pounds Pork cut into chunks
- 2 large Eggs
- 1 teaspoon Pure Sesame Oil (optional)
- 1 cup Potato Starch (or cornstarch)
- 1/2 teaspoon Sea Salt
- 1/4 teaspoon Freshly Ground Black Pepper
- 1/16 teaspoon Chinese Five Spice
- 3 Tablespoons Canola Oil
- Oil Mister

Directions:

1. In a mixing bowl, combine salt, potato starch, Chinese Five Spice, and peppers.
2. In another bowl, beat the eggs & add sesame oil.
3. Then dredge the pieces of Pork into the Potato Starch and remove the excess. Then dip each piece into the egg mixture, shake off excess, and then back into the Potato Starch mixture.
4. Place pork pieces into the Instant Pot Duo Crisp Air Fryer Basket after spray the pork with oil.
5. Close the Air Fryer lid and cook at 340°F for approximately 8 to12 minutes (or until pork is cooked), shaking the basket a couple of times for evenly distribution.
- **Nutrition Info:** Calories 521, Total Fat 21g, Total Carbs 23g, Protein 60g

166.Sweet Potato Chips

Servings: 2
Cooking Time: 40 Minutes
Ingredients:
- 2 sweet potatoes
- Salt and pepper to taste
- Olive oil
- Cinnamon

Directions:
1. Start by preheating toaster oven to 400°F.
2. Cut off each end of potato and discard.
3. Cut potatoes into 1/2-inch slices.
4. Brush a pan with olive oil and lay potato slices flat on the pan.
5. Bake for 20 minutes, then flip and bake for another 20.
- **Nutrition Info:** Calories: 139, Sodium: 29 mg, Dietary Fiber: 8.2 g, Total Fat: 0.5 g, Total Carbs: 34.1 g, Protein: 1.9 g.

167.Butter Fish With Sake And Miso

Servings: 4
Cooking Time: 11 Minutes
Ingredients:
- 4 (7-ounce) pieces of butter fish
- 1/3 cup sake
- 1/3 cup mirin
- 2/3 cup sugar
- 1 cup white miso

Directions:
1. Start by combining sake, mirin, and sugar in a sauce pan and bring to a boil.
2. Allow to boil for 5 minutes, then reduce heat and simmer for another 10 minutes.
3. Remove from heat completely and mix in miso.
4. Marinate the fish in the mixture for as long as possible, up to 3 days if possible.
5. Preheat toaster oven to 450°F and bake fish for 8 minutes.

6. Switch your setting to Broil and broil another 2-3 minutes, until the sauce is caramelized.
- **Nutrition Info:** Calories: 529, Sodium: 2892 mg, Dietary Fiber: 3.7 g, Total Fat: 5.8 g, Total Carbs: 61.9 g, Protein: 53.4 g.

168.Chicken Potato Bake

Servings: 4
Cooking Time: 25 Minutes
Ingredients:
- 4 potatoes, diced
- 1 tablespoon garlic, minced
- 1.5 tablespoons olive oil
- 1/8 teaspoon salt
- 1/8 teaspoon pepper
- 1.5 lbs. boneless skinless chicken
- 3/4 cup mozzarella cheese, shredded
- parsley chopped

Directions:
1. Toss chicken and potatoes with all the spices and oil in a baking pan.
2. Drizzle the cheese on top of the chicken and potato.
3. Press "Power Button" of Air Fry Oven and turn the dial to select the "Bake" mode.
4. Press the Time button and again turn the dial to set the cooking time to 25 minutes.
5. Now push the Temp button and rotate the dial to set the temperature at 375 degrees F.
6. Once preheated, place the baking pan inside and close its lid.
7. Serve warm.
- **Nutrition Info:** Calories 695 Total Fat 17.5 g Saturated Fat 4.8 g Cholesterol 283 mg Sodium 355 mg Total Carbs 26.4 g Fiber 1.8 g Sugar 0.8 g Protein 117.4 g

169.Lamb Gyro

Servings: 4
Cooking Time: 25 Minutes
Ingredients:
- 1 pound ground lamb
- ¼ red onion, minced
- ¼ cup mint, minced
- ¼ cup parsley, minced
- 2 cloves garlic, minced
- ½ teaspoon salt
- ⅛ teaspoon rosemary
- ½ teaspoon black pepper
- 4 slices pita bread
- ¾ cup hummus
- 1 cup romaine lettuce, shredded
- ½ onion sliced
- 1 Roma tomato, diced
- ½ cucumber, skinned and thinly sliced
- 12 mint leaves, minced
- Tzatziki sauce, to taste

Directions:

1. Mix ground lamb, red onion, mint, parsley, garlic, salt, rosemary, and black pepper until fully incorporated.
2. Select the Broil function on the COSORI Air Fryer Toaster Oven, set time to 25 minutes and temperature to 450°F, then press Start/Cancel to preheat.
3. Line the food tray with parchment paper and place ground lamb on top, shaping it into a patty 1-inch-thick and 6 inches in diameter.
4. Insert the food tray at top position in the preheated air fryer toaster oven, then press Start/Cancel.
5. Remove when done and cut into thin slices.
6. Assemble each gyro starting with pita bread, then hummus, lamb meat, lettuce, onion, tomato, cucumber, and mint leaves, then drizzle with tzatziki.
7. Serve immediately.
- **Nutrition Info:** Calories: 409 kcal Total Fat: 14.6 g Saturated Fat: 0 g Cholesterol: 0 mg Sodium: 0 mg Total Carbs: 29.9 g Fiber: 0 g Sugar: 0 g Protein: 39.4 g

170.Lemon Chicken Breasts

Servings: 4
Cooking Time: 30 Minutes
Ingredients:
- 1/4 cup olive oil
- 3 tablespoons garlic, minced
- 1/3 cup dry white wine
- 1 tablespoon lemon zest, grated
- 2 tablespoons lemon juice
- 1 1/2 teaspoons dried oregano, crushed
- 1 teaspoon thyme leaves, minced
- Salt and black pepper
- 4 skin-on boneless chicken breasts
- 1 lemon, sliced

Directions:
1. Whisk everything in a baking pan to coat the chicken breasts well.
2. Place the lemon slices on top of the chicken breasts.
3. Spread the mustard mixture over the toasted bread slices.
4. Press "Power Button" of Air Fry Oven and turn the dial to select the "Bake" mode.
5. Press the Time button and again turn the dial to set the cooking time to 30 minutes.
6. Now push the Temp button and rotate the dial to set the temperature at 370 degrees F.
7. Once preheated, place the baking pan inside and close its lid.
8. Serve warm.
- **Nutrition Info:** Calories 388 Total Fat 8 g Saturated Fat 1 g Cholesterol 153mg sodium 339 mg Total Carbs 8 g Fiber 1 g Sugar 2 g Protein 13 g

171.Parmesan Chicken Meatballs

Servings: 4
Cooking Time: 12 Minutes
Ingredients:
- 1-lb. ground chicken
- 1 large egg, beaten
- ½ cup Parmesan cheese, grated
- ½ cup pork rinds, ground
- 1 teaspoon garlic powder
- 1 teaspoon paprika
- 1 teaspoon kosher salt
- ½ teaspoon pepper
- Crust:
- ½ cup pork rinds, ground

Directions:
1. Toss all the meatball Ingredients: in a bowl and mix well.
2. Make small meatballs out this mixture and roll them in the pork rinds.
3. Place the coated meatballs in the air fryer basket.
4. Press "Power Button" of Air Fry Oven and turn the dial to select the "Bake" mode.
5. Press the Time button and again turn the dial to set the cooking time to 12 minutes.
6. Now push the Temp button and rotate the dial to set the temperature at 400 degrees F.
7. Once preheated, place the air fryer basket inside and close its lid.
8. Serve warm.
- **Nutrition Info:** Calories 529 Total Fat 17 g Saturated Fat 3 g Cholesterol 65 mg Sodium 391 mg Total Carbs 55 g Fiber 6 g Sugar 8 g Protein 41g

DINNER RECIPES

172. Green Beans And Lime Sauce

Servings: 4
Cooking Time: 20 Minutes
Ingredients:
- 1 lb. green beans, trimmed
- 2 tbsp. ghee; melted
- 1 tbsp. lime juice
- 1 tsp. chili powder
- A pinch of salt and black pepper

Directions:
1. Take a bowl and mix the ghee with the rest of the ingredients except the green beans and whisk really well.
2. Mix the green beans with the lime sauce, toss
3. Put them in your air fryer's basket and cook at 400°F for 8 minutes. Serve right away.
- **Nutrition Info:** Calories: 151; Fat: 4g; Fiber: 2g; Carbs: 4g; Protein: 6g

173. Turkey Wontons With Garlic-parmesan Sauce

Servings: 8
Cooking Time: 20 Minutes
Ingredients:
- 8 ounces cooked turkey breasts, shredded 16 wonton wrappers
- 1½ tablespoons margarine, melted
- 1/3 cup cream cheese, room temperature 8 ounces Asiago cheese, shredded
- 3 tablespoons Parmesan cheese, grated
- 1 tsp. garlic powder
- Fine sea salt and freshly ground black pepper, to taste

Directions:
1. In a small-sized bowl, mix the margarine, Parmesan, garlic powder, salt, and black pepper; give it a good stir.
2. Lightly grease a mini muffin pan; lay 1 wonton wrapper in each mini muffin cup. Fill each cup with the cream cheese and turkey mixture.
3. Air-fry for 8 minutes at 335 °F. Immediately top with Asiago cheese and serve warm.
- **Nutrition Info:** 362 Calories; 13.5g Fat; 40.4g Carbs; 18.5g Protein; 1.2g Sugars

174. Artichoke Spinach Casserole

Servings: 4
Cooking Time: 20 Minutes
Ingredients:
- ⅓cup full-fat mayonnaise
- oz. full-fat cream cheese; softened.
- ¼ cup diced yellow onion
- ⅓cup full-fat sour cream.
- ¼ cup chopped pickled jalapeños.
- 2 cups fresh spinach; chopped
- 2 cups cauliflower florets; chopped
- 1 cup artichoke hearts; chopped
- 1 tbsp. salted butter; melted.

Directions:
1. Take a large bowl, mix butter, onion, cream cheese, mayonnaise and sour cream. Fold in jalapeños, spinach, cauliflower and artichokes.
2. Pour the mixture into a 4-cup round baking dish. Cover with foil and place into the air fryer basket
3. Adjust the temperature to 370 Degrees F and set the timer for 15 minutes. In the last 2 minutes of cooking, remove the foil to brown the top. Serve warm.
- **Nutrition Info:** Calories: 423; Protein: 7g; Fiber: 3g; Fat: 33g; Carbs: 11g

175. Rigatoni With Roasted Broccoli And Chick Peas

Servings: 4
Cooking Time: 10 Minutes
Ingredients:
- 1 can anchovies packed in oil
- 4 cloves garlic, chopped
- 1 can chickpeas
- 1 chicken bouillon cube
- 1 pound broccoli, cut into small florets
- 1/2 pound whole wheat rigatoni
- 1/2 cup grated Romano cheese

Directions:
1. Drain and chop anchovies (set aside oil for later use), and cut broccoli into small florets.
2. Preheat toaster oven to 450°F.
3. In a shallow sauce pan, sauté anchovies in their oil, with garlic, until the garlic browns.
4. Drain the chickpeas, saving the canned liquid.
5. Add the chickpea liquid and bouillon to the anchovies, stir until bouillon dissolves.
6. Pour anchovy mix into a roasting pan and add broccoli and chickpeas.
7. Roast for 20 minutes.
8. While the veggies roast, cook rigatoni per package directions; drain the pasta, saving one cup of water.
9. Add the pasta to the anchovy mix and roast for another 10 minutes. Add reserved water, stirring in a little at a time until the pasta reaches the desired consistency.
10. Top with Romano and serve.
- **Nutrition Info:** Calories: 574, Sodium: 1198 mg, Dietary Fiber: 13.7 g, Total Fat: 14.0 g, Total Carbs: 81.1 g, Protein: 31.1 g.

176. Stuffed Potatoes

Servings: 4

Cooking Time: 31 Minutes
Ingredients:
- 4 potatoes, peeled
- 1 tablespoon butter
- ½ of brown onion, chopped
- 2 tablespoons chives, chopped
- ½ cup Parmesan cheese, grated
- 3 tablespoons canola oil

Directions:
1. Preheat the Air fryer to 390 ºF and grease an Air fryer basket.
2. Coat the potatoes with canola oil and arrange into the Air fryer basket.
3. Cook for about 20 minutes and transfer into a platter.
4. Cut each potato in half and scoop out the flesh from each half.
5. Heat butter in a frying pan over medium heat and add onions.
6. Sauté for about 5 minutes and dish out in a bowl.
7. Mix the onions with the potato flesh, chives, and half of cheese.
8. Stir well and stuff the potato halves evenly with the onion potato mixture.
9. Top with the remaining cheese and arrange the potato halves into the Air fryer basket.
10. Cook for about 6 minutes and dish out to serve warm.
- **Nutrition Info:** Calories: 328, Fat: 11.3g, Carbohydrates: 34.8g, Sugar: 3.1g, Protein: 5.8g, Sodium: 77mg

177.Filet Mignon With Chili Peanut Sauce

Servings: 4
Cooking Time: 20 Minutes
Ingredients:
- 2 pounds filet mignon, sliced into bite-sized strips
- 1 tablespoon oyster sauce
- 2 tablespoons sesame oil
- 2 tablespoons tamari sauce
- 1 tablespoon ginger-garlic paste
- 1 tablespoon mustard
- 1 teaspoon chili powder
- 1/4 cup peanut butter
- 2 tablespoons lime juice
- 1 teaspoon red pepper flakes
- 2 tablespoons water

Directions:
1. Place the beef strips, oyster sauce, sesame oil, tamari sauce, ginger-garlic paste, mustard, and chili powder in a large ceramic dish.
2. Cover and allow it to marinate for 2 hours in your refrigerator.
3. Cook in the preheated Air Fryer at 400 degrees F for 18 minutes, shaking the basket occasionally.

4. Mix the peanut butter with lime juice, red pepper flakes, and water. Spoon the sauce onto the air fried beef strips and serve warm.
- **Nutrition Info:** 420 Calories; 21g Fat; 5g Carbs; 50g Protein; 7g Sugars; 1g Fiber

178.Shrimps, Zucchini, And Tomatoes On The Grill

Servings: 2
Cooking Time: 15 Minutes
Ingredients:
- 10 jumbo shrimps, peeled and deveined
- Salt and pepper to taste
- 1 clove of garlic, minced
- 1 medium zucchini, sliced
- 1-pint cherry tomatoes
- ¼ cup feta cheese

Directions:
1. Place the instant pot air fryer lid on and preheat the instant pot at 390 degrees F.
2. Place the grill pan accessory in the instant pot.
3. In a mixing bowl, season the shrimps with salt and pepper. Stir in the garlic, zucchini, and tomatoes.
4. Place on the grill pan, close the air fryer lid and cook for 15 minutes.
5. Once cooked, transfer to a bowl and sprinkle with feta cheese.
- **Nutrition Info:** Calories: 257; Carbs:4.2 g; Protein: 48.9g; Fat: 5.3g

179.Bbq Pork Ribs

Servings: 2 To 3
Cooking Time: 5 Hrs 30 Minutes
Ingredients:
- 1 lb pork ribs
- 1 tsp soy sauce
- Salt and black pepper to taste
- 1 tsp oregano
- 1 tbsp + 1 tbsp maple syrup
- 3 tbsp barbecue sauce
- 2 cloves garlic, minced
- 1 tbsp cayenne pepper
- 1 tsp sesame oil

Directions:
1. Put the chops on a chopping board and use a knife to cut them into smaller pieces of desired sizes. Put them in a mixing bowl, add the soy sauce, salt, pepper, oregano, one tablespoon of maple syrup, barbecue sauce, garlic, cayenne pepper, and sesame oil. Mix well and place the pork in the fridge to marinate in the spices for 5 hours.
2. Preheat the Air Fryer to 350 F. Open the Air Fryer and place the ribs in the fryer basket. Slide the fryer basket in and cook for 15 minutes. Open the Air fryer, turn the ribs

using tongs, apply the remaining maple syrup with a brush, close the Air Fryer, and continue cooking for 10 minutes.

- **Nutrition Info:** 346 Calories; 11g Fat; 4g Carbs; 32g Protein; 1g Sugars; 1g Fiber

180. Buttered Scallops

Servings: 2
Cooking Time: 4 Minutes
Ingredients:

- ¾ pound sea scallops, cleaned and patted very dry
- 1 tablespoon butter, melted
- ½ tablespoon fresh thyme, minced
- Salt and black pepper, as required

Directions:

1. Preheat the Air fryer to 390 degree F and grease an Air fryer basket.
2. Mix scallops, butter, thyme, salt, and black pepper in a bowl.
3. Arrange scallops in the Air fryer basket and cook for about 4 minutes.
4. Dish out the scallops in a platter and serve hot.
- **Nutrition Info:** Calories: 202, Fat: 7.1g, Carbohydrates: 4.4g, Sugar: 0g, Protein: 28.7g, Sodium: 393mg

181. Shrimp Scampi

Servings: 6
Cooking Time: 7 Minutes
Ingredients:

- 4 tablespoons salted butter
- 1 pound shrimp, peeled and deveined
- 2 tablespoons fresh basil, chopped
- 1 tablespoon fresh chives, chopped
- 1 tablespoon fresh lemon juice
- 1 tablespoon garlic, minced
- 2 teaspoons red pepper flakes, crushed
- 2 tablespoons dry white wine

Directions:

1. Preheat the Air fryer to 325 ºF and grease an Air fryer pan.
2. Heat butter, lemon juice, garlic, and red pepper flakes in a pan and return the pan to Air fryer basket.
3. Cook for about 2 minutes and stir in shrimp, basil, chives and wine.
4. Cook for about 5 minutes and dish out the mixture onto serving plates.
5. Serve hot.
- **Nutrition Info:** Calories: 250, Fat: 13.7g, Carbohydrates: 3.3g, Sugar: 0.3g, Protein: 26.3g, Sodium: 360mg

182. Tex-mex Chicken Quesadillas

Servings: 4
Cooking Time: 10 Minutes
Ingredients:

- 2 green onions
- 2 cups shredded skinless rotisserie chicken meat
- 1-1/2 cups shredded Monterey Jack cheese
- 1 pickled jalapeño
- 1/4 cup fresh cilantro leaves
- 4 burrito-size flour tortillas
- 1/2 cup reduced-fat sour cream

Directions:

1. Start by preheating toaster oven to 425°F.
2. Thinly slice the green onions and break apart.
3. Mix together chicken, cheese, jalapeño, and onions in a bowl, then evenly divide mixture onto one half of each tortilla.
4. Fold opposite half over mixture and place quesadillas onto a baking sheet.
5. Bake for 10 minutes.
6. Cut in halves or quarters and serve with sour cream.
- **Nutrition Info:** Calories: 830, Sodium: 921 mg, Dietary Fiber: 1.8 g, Total Fat: 59.0 g, Total Carbs: 13.8 g, Protein: 60.8 g.

183. Salmon Steak Grilled With Cilantro Garlic Sauce

Servings: 2
Cooking Time: 15 Minutes
Ingredients:

- 2 salmon steaks
- Salt and pepper to taste
- 2 tablespoons vegetable oil
- 2 cloves of garlic, minced
- 1 cup cilantro leaves
- ½ cup Greek yogurt
- 1 teaspoon honey

Directions:

1. Place the instant pot air fryer lid on and preheat the instant pot at 390 degrees F.
2. Place the grill pan accessory in the instant pot.
3. Season the salmon steaks with salt and pepper. Brush with oil.
4. Place on the grill pan, close the air fryer lid and grill for 15 minutes and make sure to flip halfway through the cooking time.
5. In a food processor, mix the garlic, cilantro leaves, yogurt, and honey. Season with salt and pepper to taste. Pulse until smooth.
6. Serve the salmon steaks with the cilantro sauce.
- **Nutrition Info:** Calories: 485; Carbs: 6.3g; Protein: 47.6g; Fat: 29.9g

184. Amazing Bacon And Potato Platter

Servings: 4
Cooking Time: 40 Minutes
Ingredients:

- 4 potatoes, halved

- 6 garlic cloves, squashed
- 4 streaky cut rashers bacon
- 2 sprigs rosemary
- 1 tbsp olive oil

Directions:

1. Preheat your air fryer to 392 f. In a mixing bowl, mix garlic, bacon, potatoes and rosemary; toss in oil. Place the mixture in your air fryer's cooking basket and roast for 25-30 minutes. Serve and enjoy!
- **Nutrition Info:** Calories: 336 Cal Total Fat: 18.5 g Saturated Fat: 0 g Cholesterol: 82 mg Sodium: 876 mg Total Carbs: 69.9 g Fiber: 0 g Sugar: 0 g Protein: 0 g

185.Corned Beef With Carrots

Servings: 3
Cooking Time: 35 Minutes
Ingredients:

- 1 tbsp beef spice
- 1 whole onion, chopped
- 4 carrots, chopped
- 12 oz bottle beer
- 1½ cups chicken broth
- 4 pounds corned beef

Directions:

1. Preheat your air fryer to 380 f. Cover beef with beer and set aside for 20 minutes. Place carrots, onion and beef in a pot and heat over high heat. Add in broth and bring to a boil. Drain boiled meat and veggies; set aside.
2. Top with beef spice. Place the meat and veggies in your air fryer's cooking basket and cook for 30 minutes.
- **Nutrition Info:** Calories: 464 Cal Total Fat: 17 g Saturated Fat: 6.8 g Cholesterol: 91.7 mg Sodium: 1904.2 mg Total Carbs: 48.9 g Fiber: 7.2 g Sugar: 5.8 g Protein: 30.6 g

186.Miso-glazed Salmon

Servings: 4
Cooking Time: 5 Minutes
Ingredients:

- 1/4 cup red or white miso
- 1/3 cup sake
- 1 tablespoon soy sauce
- 2 tablespoons vegetable oil
- 1/4 cup sugar
- 4 skinless salmon filets

Directions:

1. In a shallow bowl, mix together the miso, sake, oil, soy sauce, and sugar.
2. Toss the salmon in the mixture until thoroughly coated on all sides.
3. Preheat your toaster oven to "high" on broil mode.

4. Place salmon in a broiling pan and broil until the top is well charred—about 5 minutes.
- **Nutrition Info:** Calories: 401, Sodium: 315 mg, Dietary Fiber: 0 g, Total Fat: 19.2 g, Total Carbs: 14.1 g, Protein: 39.2 g.

187.Almond Asparagus

Servings: 3
Cooking Time: 6 Minutes
Ingredients:

- 1 pound asparagus
- 1/3 cup almonds, sliced
- 2 tablespoons olive oil
- 2 tablespoons balsamic vinegar
- Salt and black pepper, to taste

Directions:

1. Preheat the Air fryer to 400 ºF and grease an Air fryer basket.
2. Mix asparagus, oil, vinegar, salt, and black pepper in a bowl and toss to coat well.
3. Arrange asparagus into the Air fryer basket and sprinkle with the almond slices.
4. Cook for about 6 minutes and dish out to serve hot.
- **Nutrition Info:** Calories: 173, Fat: 14.8g, Carbohydrates: 8.2g, Sugar: 3.3g, Protein: 5.6g, Sodium: 54mg

188.Prawn Burgers

Servings: 2
Cooking Time: 6 Minutes
Ingredients:

- ½ cup prawns, peeled, deveined and finely chopped
- ½ cup breadcrumbs
- 2-3 tablespoons onion, finely chopped
- 3 cups fresh baby greens
- ½ teaspoon ginger, minced
- ½ teaspoon garlic, minced
- ½ teaspoon red chili powder
- ½ teaspoon ground cumin
- ¼ teaspoon ground turmeric
- Salt and ground black pepper, as required

Directions:

1. Preheat the Air fryer to 390 degree F and grease an Air fryer basket.
2. Mix the prawns, breadcrumbs, onion, ginger, garlic, and spices in a bowl.
3. Make small-sized patties from the mixture and transfer to the Air fryer basket.
4. Cook for about 6 minutes and dish out in a platter.
5. Serve immediately warm alongside the baby greens.
- **Nutrition Info:** Calories: 240, Fat: 2.7g, Carbohydrates: 37.4g, Sugar: 4g, Protein: 18g, Sodium: 371mg

189.Fish Cakes With Horseradish Sauce

Servings: 4
Cooking Time: 20 Minutes
Ingredients:
- Halibut Cakes:
- 1 pound halibut
- 2 tablespoons olive oil
- 1/2 teaspoon cayenne pepper
- 1/4 teaspoon black pepper
- Salt, to taste
- 2 tablespoons cilantro, chopped
- 1 shallot, chopped
- 2 garlic cloves, minced
- 1 cup Romano cheese, grated
- 1 egg, whisked
- 1 tablespoon Worcestershire sauce
- Mayo Sauce:
- 1 teaspoon horseradish, grated
- 1/2 cup mayonnaise

Directions:
1. Start by preheating your Air Fryer to 380 degrees F. Spritz the Air Fryer basket with cooking oil.
2. Mix all ingredients for the halibut cakes in a bowl; knead with your hands until everything is well incorporated.
3. Shape the mixture into equally sized patties. Transfer your patties to the Air Fryer basket. Cook the fish patties for 10 minutes, turning them over halfway through.
4. Mix the horseradish and mayonnaise. Serve the halibut cakes with the horseradish mayo.
- **Nutrition Info:** 532 Calories; 32g Fat; 3g Carbs; 28g Protein; 3g Sugars; 6g Fiber

190.Adobe Turkey Chimichangas

Servings: 4
Cooking Time: 15 Minutes
Ingredients:
- 1 pound thickly-sliced smoked turkey from deli counter, chopped
- 1 tablespoon chili powder
- 2 cups shredded slaw cabbage
- 1 to 2 chipotles in adobo sauce
- 1 cup tomato sauce
- 3 chopped scallions
- Salt and pepper
- 4 (12-inch) flour tortillas
- 1-1/2 cups pepper jack cheese
- 2 tablespoons olive oil
- 1 cup sour cream
- 2 tablespoons chopped cilantro

Directions:
1. Start by preheating toaster oven to 400°F.
2. In a medium bowl mix together turkey and chili powder.

3. Add cabbage, chipotles, tomato sauce, and scallions; mix well.
4. Season cabbage mixture with salt and pepper and turn a few times.
5. Warm tortillas in a microwave or on a stove top.
6. Lay cheese flat in each tortilla and top with turkey mixture.
7. Fold in the top and bottom of the tortilla, then roll to close.
8. Brush baking tray with oil, then place chimichangas on tray and brush with oil.
9. Bake for 15 minutes or until tortilla is golden brown.
10. Top with sour cream and cilantro and serve.
- **Nutrition Info:** Calories: 638, Sodium: 1785 mg, Dietary Fiber: 4.2 g, Total Fat: 44.0 g, Total Carbs: 23.9 g, Protein: 38.4 g.

191.Cheddar & Dijon Tuna Melt

Servings: 1
Cooking Time: 7 Minutes
Ingredients:
- 1 (6-ounce) can tuna, drained and flaked
- 2 tablespoons mayonnaise
- 1 pinch salt
- 1 teaspoon balsamic vinegar
- 1 teaspoon Dijon mustard
- 2 slices whole wheat bread
- 2 teaspoons chopped dill pickle
- 1/4 cup shredded sharp cheddar cheese

Directions:
1. Start by preheating toaster oven to 375°F.
2. Put bread in toaster while it warms.
3. Mix together tuna, mayo, salt, vinegar, mustard, and pickle in a small bowl.
4. Remove bread from oven and put tuna mixture on one side and the cheese on the other.
5. Return to toaster oven and bake for 7 minutes.
6. Combine slices, then cut and serve.
- **Nutrition Info:** Calories: 688, Sodium: 1024 mg, Dietary Fiber: 4.1 g, Total Fat: 35.0 g, Total Carbs: 31.0 g, Protein: 59.9 g.

192.Air Fryer Veggie Quesdillas

Servings: 4
Cooking Time: 40 Minutes
Ingredients:
- 4 sprouted whole-grain flour tortillas (6-in.)
- 1 cup sliced red bell pepper
- 4 ounces reduced-fat Cheddar cheese, shredded
- 1 cup sliced zucchini
- 1 cup canned black beans, drained and rinsed (no salt)
- Cooking spray
- 2 ounces plain 2% reduced-fat Greek yogurt

- 1 teaspoon lime zest
- 1 Tbsp. fresh juice (from 1 lime)
- ¼ tsp. ground cumin
- 2 tablespoons chopped fresh cilantro
- 1/2 cup drained refrigerated pico de gallo

Directions:
1. Place tortillas on work surface, sprinkle 2 tablespoons shredded cheese over half of each tortilla and top with cheese on each tortilla with 1/4 cup each red pepper slices, zucchini slices, and black beans. Sprinkle evenly with remaining 1/2 cup cheese.
2. Fold tortillas over to form half-moon shaped quesadillas, lightly coat with cooking spray, and secure with toothpicks.
3. Lightly spray air fryer basket with cooking spray. Place 2 quesadillas in the basket, and cook at 400°F for 10 minutes until tortillas are golden brown and slightly crispy, cheese is melted, and vegetables are slightly softened. Turn quesadillas over halfway through cooking.
4. Repeat with remaining quesadillas.
5. Meanwhile, stir yogurt, lime juice, lime zest and cumin in a small bowl.
6. Cut each quesadilla into wedges and sprinkle with cilantro.
7. Serve with 1 tablespoon cumin cream and 2 tablespoons pico de gallo each.
- **Nutrition Info:** Calories 291 Fat 8g Saturated fat 4g Unsaturated fat 3g Protein 17g Carbohydrate 36g Fiber 8g Sugars 3g Sodium 518mg Calcium 30% DV Potassium 6% DV

193.Spicy Cauliflower Rice

Servings: 2
Cooking Time: 22 Minutes
Ingredients:
- 1 cauliflower head, cut into florets 1/2 tsp cumin
- 1/2 tsp chili powder
- 6 onion spring, chopped 2 jalapenos, chopped
- 4 tbsp olive oil
- 1 zucchini, trimmed and cut into cubes 1/2 tsp paprika
- 1/2 tsp garlic powder 1/2 tsp cayenne pepper 1/2 tsp pepper
- 1/2 tsp salt

Directions:
1. Preheat the air fryer to 370 F.
2. Add cauliflower florets into the food processor and process until it looks like rice.
3. Transfer cauliflower rice into the air fryer baking pan and drizzle with half oil.
4. Place pan in the air fryer and cook for 12 minutes, stir halfway through.

5. Heat remaining oil in a small pan over medium heat.
6. Add zucchini and cook for 5-8 minutes.
7. Add onion and jalapenos and cook for 5 minutes.
8. Add spices and stir well. Set aside.
9. Add cauliflower rice in the zucchini mixture and stir well.
10. Serve and enjoy.
- **Nutrition Info:** Calories 254 Fat 28 g Carbohydrates 12.3 g Sugar 5 g

194.Mozzarella & Olive Pizza Bagels

Servings: 4
Cooking Time: 10 Minutes
Ingredients:
- 2 whole wheat bagels
- 1/4 cup marinara sauce
- 1/4 teaspoon Italian seasoning
- 1/8 teaspoon red pepper flakes
- 3/4 cup shredded low-moisture mozzarella cheese
- 1/4 cup chopped green pepper
- 3 tablespoons sliced black olives
- Fresh basil
- 1 teaspoon parmesan cheese

Directions:
1. Start by preheating toaster oven to 375°F and lining a pan with parchment paper.
2. Cut bagels in half and lay on pan with inside facing up. Spread sauce over each half.
3. Sprinkle red pepper flakes and 2 tablespoons of mozzarella over each half.
4. Top each half with olives and peppers and then top with another tablespoon of mozzarella.
5. Bake for 8 minutes, then switch to broil setting and broil for another 2 minutes. Top with basil and parmesan and serve.
- **Nutrition Info:** Calories: 222, Sodium: 493 mg, Dietary Fiber: 1.9 g, Total Fat: 6.1 g, Total Carbs: 30.2 g, Protein: 12.1 g.

195.Pepper Pork Chops

Servings: 2
Cooking Time: 6 Minutes
Ingredients:
- 2 pork chops
- 1 egg white
- ¾ cup xanthum gum
- ½ teaspoon sea salt
- ¼ teaspoon freshly ground black pepper
- 1 oil mister

Directions:
1. Preheat the Air fryer to 400 degree F and grease an Air fryer basket.
2. Whisk egg white with salt and black pepper in a bowl and dip the pork chops in it.

3. Cover the bowl and marinate for about 20 minutes.
4. Pour the xanthum gum over both sides of the chops and spray with oil mister.
5. Arrange the chops in the Air fryer basket and cook for about 6 minutes.
6. Dish out in a bowl and serve warm.
- **Nutrition Info:** Calories: 541, Fat: 34g, Carbohydrates: 3.4g, Sugar: 1g, Protein: 20.3g, Sodium: 547mg

196.Cheese Zucchini Boats

Servings: 2
Cooking Time: 20 Minutes
Ingredients:
- 2 medium zucchinis
- ¼ cup full-fat ricotta cheese
- ¼ cup shredded mozzarella cheese
- ¼ cup low-carb, no-sugar-added pasta sauce.
- 2 tbsp. grated vegetarian Parmesan cheese
- 1 tbsp. avocado oil
- ¼ tsp. garlic powder.
- ½ tsp. dried parsley.
- ¼ tsp. dried oregano.

Directions:
1. Cut off 1-inch from the top and bottom of each zucchini.
2. Slice zucchini in half lengthwise and use a spoon to scoop out a bit of the inside, making room for filling. Brush with oil and spoon 2 tbsp. pasta sauce into each shell
3. Take a medium bowl, mix ricotta, mozzarella, oregano, garlic powder and parsley
4. Spoon the mixture into each zucchini shell. Place stuffed zucchini shells into the air fryer basket.
5. Adjust the temperature to 350 Degrees F and set the timer for 20 minutes
6. To remove from the fryer basket, use tongs or a spatula and carefully lift out. Top with Parmesan. Serve immediately.
- **Nutrition Info:** Calories: 215; Protein: 15g; Fiber: 7g; Fat: 19g; Carbs: 3g

197.Baby Portabellas With Romano Cheese

Servings: 4
Cooking Time: 20 Minutes
Ingredients:
- 1 pound baby portabellas
- 1/2 cup almond meal
- 2 eggs
- 2 tablespoons milk
- 1 cup Romano cheese, grated
- Sea salt and ground black pepper
- 1/2 teaspoon shallot powder
- 1 teaspoon garlic powder

- 1/2 teaspoon cumin powder
- 1/2 teaspoon cayenne pepper

Directions:
1. Pat the mushrooms dry with a paper towel.
2. To begin, set up your breading station. Place the almond meal in a shallow dish. In a separate dish, whisk the eggs with milk.
3. Finally, place grated Romano cheese and seasonings in the third dish.
4. Start by dredging the baby portabellas in the almond meal mixture; then, dip them into the egg wash. Press the baby portabellas into Romano cheese, coating evenly.
5. Spritz the Air Fryer basket with cooking oil. Add the baby portabellas and cook at 400 degrees F for 6 minutes, flipping them halfway through the cooking time.
- **Nutrition Info:** 230 Calories; 13g Fat; 2g Carbs; 11g Protein; 8g Sugars; 6g Fiber

198.Oven-fried Herbed Chicken

Servings: 2
Cooking Time: 15 Minutes
Ingredients:
- 1/2 cup buttermilk
- 2 cloves garlic, minced
- 1-1/2 teaspoons salt
- 1 tablespoon oil
- 1/2 pound boneless, skinless chicken breasts
- 1 cup rolled oats
- 1/2 teaspoon red pepper flakes
- 1/2 cup grated parmesan cheese
- 1/4 cup fresh basil leaves or rosemary needles
- Olive oil spray

Directions:
1. Mix together buttermilk, oil, 1/2 teaspoon salt, and garlic in a shallow bowl.
2. Roll chicken in buttermilk and refrigerate in bowl overnight.
3. Preheat your toaster oven to 425°F.
4. Mix together the oats, red pepper, salt, parmesan, and basil, and mix roughly to break up oats.
5. Place the mixture on a plate.
6. Remove the chicken from the buttermilk mixture and let any excess drip off.
7. Roll the chicken in the oat mixture and transfer to a baking sheet lightly coated with olive oil spray.
8. Spray the chicken with oil spray and bake for 15 minutes.
- **Nutrition Info:** Calories: 651, Sodium: 713 mg, Dietary Fiber: 4.4 g, Total Fat: 31.2 g, Total Carbs: 34.1 g, Protein: 59.5 g.

199.Easy Air Fryed Roasted Asparagus

Servings: 4
Cooking Time: 10 Minutes
Ingredients:
- 1 bunch fresh asparagus
- 1 ½ tsp herbs de provence
- Fresh lemon wedge (optional)
- 1 tablespoon olive oil or cooking spray
- Salt and pepper to taste

Directions:
1. Wash asparagus and trim off hard ends
2. Drizzle asparagus with olive oil and add seasonings
3. Place asparagus in air fryer and cook on 360F for 6 to 10 minutes
4. Drizzle squeezed lemon over roasted asparagus.
- **Nutrition Info:** Calories 46 protein 2g fat 3g net carbs 1g

200.Paprika Crab Burgers

Servings: 3
Cooking Time: 20 Minutes
Ingredients:
- 2 eggs, beaten
- 1 shallot, chopped
- 2 garlic cloves, crushed
- 1 tablespoon olive oil
- 1 teaspoon yellow mustard
- 1 teaspoon fresh cilantro, chopped
- 10 ounces crab meat
- 1 teaspoon smoked paprika
- 1/2 teaspoon ground black pepper
- Sea salt, to taste
- 3/4 cup parmesan cheese

Directions:
1. In a mixing bowl, thoroughly combine the eggs, shallot, garlic, olive oil, mustard, cilantro, crab meat, paprika, black pepper, and salt. Mix until well combined.
2. Shape the mixture into 6 patties. Roll the crab patties over grated parmesan cheese, coating well on all sides. Place in your refrigerator for 2 hours.
3. Spritz the crab patties with cooking oil on both sides. Cook in the preheated Air Fryer at 360 degrees F for 14 minutes. Serve on dinner rolls if desired.
- **Nutrition Info:** 279 Calories; 14g Fat; 7g Carbs; 23g Protein; 5g Sugars; 6g Fiber

201.Tomato Stuffed Pork Roll

Servings: 4
Cooking Time: 15 Minutes
Ingredients:
- 1 scallion, chopped
- ¼ cup sun-dried tomatoes, chopped finely
- 2 tablespoons fresh parsley, chopped
- 4: 6-ouncepork cutlets, pounded slightly
- Salt and freshly ground black pepper, to taste
- 2 teaspoons paprika
- ½ tablespoon olive oil

Directions:
1. Preheat the Air fryer to 390 degree F and grease an Air fryer basket.
2. Mix scallion, tomatoes, parsley, salt and black pepper in a bowl.
3. Coat each cutlet with tomato mixture and roll up the cutlet, securing with cocktail sticks.
4. Coat the rolls with oil and rub with paprika, salt and black pepper.
5. Arrange the rolls in the Air fryer basket and cook for about 15 minutes, flipping once in between.
6. Dish out in a platter and serve warm.
- **Nutrition Info:** Calories: 244, Fat: 14.5g, Carbohydrates: 20.1g, Sugar: 1.7g, Protein: 8.2g, Sodium: 670mg

202.Cheese Breaded Pork

Servings: 6
Cooking Time: 15 Minutes
Ingredients:
- 6 pork chops
- 6 tbsp seasoned breadcrumbs
- 2 tbsp parmesan cheese, grated
- 1 tbsp melted butter
- ½ cup mozzarella cheese, shredded
- 1 tbsp marinara sauce

Directions:
1. Preheat your air fryer to 390 f. Grease the cooking basket with cooking spray. In a small bowl, mix breadcrumbs and parmesan cheese. In another microwave proof bowl, add butter and melt in the microwave.
2. Brush the pork with butter and dredge into the breadcrumbs. Add pork to the cooking basket and cook for 6 minutes. Turnover and top with marinara sauce and shredded mozzarella; cook for 3 more minutes
- **Nutrition Info:** Calories: 431 Cal Total Fat: 0 g Saturated Fat: 0 g Cholesterol: 0 mg Sodium: 0 mg Total Carbs: 0 g Fiber: 0 g Sugar: 0 g Protein: 0 g

203.Sesame Mustard Greens

Servings: 4
Cooking Time: 11 Minutes
Ingredients:
- 2 garlic cloves, minced
- 1 pound mustard greens, torn
- 1 tablespoon olive oil
- ½ cup yellow onion, sliced
- Salt and black pepper to the taste

- 3 tablespoons veggie stock
- ¼ teaspoon dark sesame oil

Directions:
1. Heat up a pan that fits your air fryer with the oil over medium heat, add onions, stir and brown them for 5 minutes.
2. Add garlic, stock, greens, salt and pepper, stir, introduce in your air fryer and cook at 350 °F for 6 minutes.
3. Add sesame oil, toss to coat, divide among plates and serve.
- **Nutrition Info:** Calories: 173; Fat: 6g; Fiber: 2g; Carbs: 4g; Protein: 5g

204.Greek-style Monkfish With Vegetables

Servings: 2
Cooking Time: 20 Minutes
Ingredients:
- 2 teaspoons olive oil
- 1 cup celery, sliced
- 2 bell peppers, sliced
- 1 teaspoon dried thyme
- 1/2 teaspoon dried marjoram
- 1/2 teaspoon dried rosemary
- 2 monkfish fillets
- 1 tablespoon soy sauce
- 2 tablespoons lime juice
- Coarse salt and ground black pepper, to taste
- 1 teaspoon cayenne pepper
- 1/2 cup Kalamata olives, pitted and sliced

Directions:
1. In a nonstick skillet, heat the olive oil for 1 minute. Once hot, sauté the celery and peppers until tender, about 4 minutes. Sprinkle with thyme, marjoram, and rosemary and set aside.
2. Toss the fish fillets with the soy sauce, lime juice, salt, black pepper, and cayenne pepper. Place the fish fillets in a lightly greased cooking basket and bake at 390 degrees F for 8 minutes.
3. Turn them over, add the olives, and cook an additional 4 minutes. Serve with the sautéed vegetables on the side.
- **Nutrition Info:** 292 Calories; 11g Fat; 1g Carbs; 22g Protein; 9g Sugars; 6g Fiber

205.Lemon Garlic Shrimps

Servings: 2
Cooking Time: 8 Minutes
Ingredients:
- ¾ pound medium shrimp, peeled and deveined
- 1½ tablespoons fresh lemon juice
- 1 tablespoon olive oil
- 1 teaspoon lemon pepper
- ¼ teaspoon paprika
- ¼ teaspoon garlic powder

Directions:
1. Preheat the Air fryer to 400 degree F and grease an Air fryer basket.
2. Mix lemon juice, olive oil, lemon pepper, paprika and garlic powder in a large bowl.
3. Stir in the shrimp and toss until well combined.
4. Arrange shrimp into the Air fryer basket in a single layer and cook for about 8 minutes.
5. Dish out the shrimp in serving plates and serve warm.
- **Nutrition Info:** Calories: 260, Fat: 12.4g, Carbohydrates: 0.3g, Sugar: 0.1g, Protein: 35.6g, Sodium: 619mg

206.Shrimp Casserole Louisiana Style

Servings: 2
Cooking Time: 35 Minutes
Ingredients:
- 3/4 cup uncooked instant rice
- 3/4 cup water
- 1/2 pound small shrimp, peeled and deveined
- 1 tablespoon butter
- 1/2 (4 ounces) can sliced mushrooms, drained
- 1/2 (8 ounces) container sour cream
- 1/3 cup shredded Cheddar cheese

Directions:
1. Place the instant pot air fryer lid on, lightly grease baking pan of the instant pot with cooking spray. Add rice, water, mushrooms, and butter. Cover with foil and place the baking pan in the instant pot.
2. Close the air fryer lid and cook at 360 ºF for 20 minutes.
3. Open foil cover, stir in shrimps, return foil and let it rest for 5 minutes.
4. Remove foil completely and stir in sour cream. Mix well and evenly spread rice. Top with cheese.
5. Cook for 7 minutes at 390 ºF until tops are lightly browned.
6. Serve and enjoy.
- **Nutrition Info:** Calories: 569; Carbs: 38.5g; Protein: 31.8g; Fat: 31.9g

207.Party Stuffed Pork Chops

Servings: 4
Cooking Time: 40 Minutes
Ingredients:
- 8 pork chops
- ¼ tsp pepper
- 4 cups stuffing mix
- ½ tsp salt
- 2 tbsp olive oil
- 4 garlic cloves, minced
- 2 tbsp sage leaves

Directions:

1. Preheat your air fryer to 350 f. cut a hole in pork chops and fill chops with stuffing mix. In a bowl, mix sage leaves, garlic cloves, oil, salt and pepper. Cover chops with marinade and let marinate for 10 minutes. Place the chops in your air fryer's cooking basket and cook for 25 minutes. Serve and enjoy!
- **Nutrition Info:** Calories: 364 Cal Total Fat: 13 g Saturated Fat: 4 g Cholesterol: 119 mg Sodium: 349 mg Total Carbs: 19 g Fiber: 3 g Sugar: 6 g Protein: 40 g

208.Five Spice Pork

Servings: 4
Cooking Time: 20 Minutes
Ingredients:
- 1-pound pork belly
- 2 tablespoons swerve
- 2 tablespoons dark soy sauce
- 1 tablespoon Shaoxing: cooking wine
- 2 teaspoons garlic, minced
- 2 teaspoons ginger, minced
- 1 tablespoon hoisin sauce
- 1 teaspoon Chinese Five Spice

Directions:
1. Preheat the Air fryer to 390 degree F and grease an Air fryer basket.
2. Mix all the ingredients in a bowl and place in the Ziplock bag.
3. Seal the bag, shake it well and refrigerate to marinate for about 1 hour.
4. Remove the pork from the bag and arrange it in the Air fryer basket.
5. Cook for about 15 minutes and dish out in a bowl to serve warm.
- **Nutrition Info:** Calories: 604, Fat: 30.6g, Carbohydrates: 1.4g, Sugar: 20.3g, Protein: 19.8g, Sodium: 834mg

209.Traditional English Fish And Chips

Servings: 4
Cooking Time: 17 Minutes
Ingredients:
- 1 3/4 pounds potatoes
- 4 tablespoons olive oil
- 1-1/4 teaspoons kosher salt
- 1-1/4 teaspoons black pepper
- 8 sprigs fresh thyme
- 4 (6-ounce) pieces cod
- 1 lemon
- 1 clove garlic
- 2 tablespoons capers

Directions:
1. Start by preheating toaster oven to 450°F.
2. Cut potatoes into 1-inch chunks.
3. Place potatoes, 2 tablespoons oil, salt, and thyme in a baking tray and toss to combine.
4. Spread in a flat layer and bake for 30 minutes.

5. Wrap mixture in foil to keep warm.
6. Wipe tray with a paper towel and then lay cod in the tray.
7. Slice the lemon and top cod with lemon, salt, pepper, and thyme.
8. Drizzle rest of the oil over the cod and bake for 12 minutes.
9. Place cod and potatoes on separate pans and bake together for an additional 5 minutes.
10. Combine and serve.
- **Nutrition Info:** Calories: 442, Sodium: 1002 mg, Dietary Fiber: 5.4 g, Total Fat: 15.8 g, Total Carbs: 32.7 g, Protein: 42.5 g.

210.Garlic Lamb Shank

Servings: 5
Cooking Time: 24 Minutes
Ingredients:
- 17 oz. lamb shanks
- 2 tablespoon garlic, peeled
- 1 teaspoon kosher salt
- 1 tablespoon dried parsley
- 4 oz chive stems, chopped
- ½ cup chicken stock
- 1 teaspoon butter
- 1 teaspoon dried rosemary
- 1 teaspoon nutmeg
- ½ teaspoon ground black pepper

Directions:
1. Chop the garlic roughly.
2. Make the cuts in the lamb shank and fill the cuts with the chopped garlic.
3. Then sprinkle the lamb shank with the kosher salt, dried parsley, dried rosemary, nutmeg, and ground black pepper.
4. Stir the spices on the lamb shank gently.
5. Then put the butter and chicken stock in the air fryer basket tray.
6. Preheat the air fryer to 380 F.
7. Put the chives in the air fryer basket tray.
8. Add the lamb shank and cook the meat for 24 minutes.
9. When the lamb shank is cooked – transfer it to the serving plate and sprinkle with the remaining liquid from the cooked meat.
10. Enjoy!
- **Nutrition Info:** calories 205, fat 8.2, fiber 0.8, carbs 3.8, protein 27.2

211.Beef Pieces With Tender Broccoli

Servings: 4
Cooking Time: 13 Minutes
Ingredients:
- 6 oz. broccoli
- 10 oz. beef brisket
- 4 oz chive stems
- 1 teaspoon paprika
- 1/3 cup water

- 1 teaspoon olive oil
- 1 teaspoon butter
- 1 tablespoon flax seeds
- ½ teaspoon chili flakes

Directions:
1. Cut the beef brisket into the medium/convenient pieces.
2. Sprinkle the beef pieces with the paprika and chili flakes.
3. Mix the meat up with the help of the hands.
4. Then preheat the air fryer to 360 F.
5. Spray the air fryer basket tray with the olive oil.
6. Put the beef pieces in the air fryer basket tray and cook the meat for 7 minutes.
7. Stir it once during the cooking.
8. Meanwhile, separate the broccoli into the florets.
9. When the time is over – add the broccoli florets in the air fryer basket tray.
10. Sprinkle the ingredients with the flax seeds and butter.
11. Add water.
12. Dice the chives and add them in the air fryer basket tray too.
13. Stir it gently using the wooden spatula.
14. Then cook the dish at 265 F for 6 minutes more.
15. When the broccoli is tender – the dish is cooked.
16. Serve the dish little bit chilled.
17. Enjoy!
- **Nutrition Info:** calories 187, fat 7.3, fiber 2.4, carbs 6.2, protein 23.4

212.Pollock With Kalamata Olives And Capers

Servings: 3
Cooking Time: 20 Minutes
Ingredients:
- 2 tablespoons olive oil
- 1 red onion, sliced
- 2 cloves garlic, chopped
- 1 Florina pepper, deveined and minced
- 3 pollock fillets,skinless
- 2 ripe tomatoes, diced
- 12 Kalamata olives, pitted and chopped
- 2 tablespoons capers
- 1 teaspoon oregano
- 1 teaspoon rosemary
- Sea salt, to taste
- 1/2 cup white wine

Directions:
1. Start by preheating your Air Fryer to 360 degrees F. Heat the oil in a baking pan. Once hot, sauté the onion, garlic, and pepper for 2 to 3 minutes or until fragrant.
2. Add the fish fillets to the baking pan. Top with the tomatoes, olives, and capers.

Sprinkle with the oregano, rosemary, and salt. Pour in white wine and transfer to the cooking basket.
3. Turn the temperature to 395 degrees F and bake for 10 minutes. Taste for seasoning and serve on individual plates, garnished with some extra Mediterranean herbs if desired. Enjoy!
- **Nutrition Info:** 480 Calories; 37g Fat; 9g Carbs; 49g Protein; 5g Sugars; 2g Fiber

213.Homemade Beef Stroganoff

Servings: 3
Cooking Time: 20 Minutes
Ingredients:
- 1 pound thin steak
- 4 tbsp butter
- 1 whole onion, chopped
- 1 cup sour cream
- 8 oz mushrooms, sliced
- 4 cups beef broth
- 16 oz egg noodles, cooked

Directions:
1. Preheat your Air Fryer to 400 F. Using a microwave proof bowl, melt butter in a microwave oven. In a mixing bowl, mix the melted butter, sliced mushrooms, cream, onion, and beef broth.
2. Pour the mixture over steak and set aside for 10 minutes. Place the marinated beef in your fryer's cooking basket, and cook for 10 minutes. Serve with cooked egg noodles and enjoy!
- **Nutrition Info:** 456 Calories; 37g Fat; 1g Carbs; 21g Protein; 5g Sugars; 6g Fiber

214.Roasted Garlic Zucchini Rolls

Servings: 4
Cooking Time: 20 Minutes
Ingredients:
- 2 medium zucchinis
- ½ cup full-fat ricotta cheese
- ¼ white onion; peeled. And diced
- 2 cups spinach; chopped
- ¼ cup heavy cream
- ½ cup sliced baby portobello mushrooms
- ¾ cup shredded mozzarella cheese, divided.
- 2 tbsp. unsalted butter.
- 2 tbsp. vegetable broth.
- ½ tsp. finely minced roasted garlic
- ¼ tsp. dried oregano.
- ⅛ tsp. xanthan gum
- ¼ tsp. salt
- ½ tsp. garlic powder.

Directions:
1. Using a mandoline or sharp knife, slice zucchini into long strips lengthwise. Place strips between paper towels to absorb moisture. Set aside

2. In a medium saucepan over medium heat, melt butter. Add onion and sauté until fragrant. Add garlic and sauté 30 seconds.
3. Pour in heavy cream, broth and xanthan gum. Turn off heat and whisk mixture until it begins to thicken, about 3 minutes.
4. Take a medium bowl, add ricotta, salt, garlic powder and oregano and mix well. Fold in spinach, mushrooms and ½ cup mozzarella
5. Pour half of the sauce into a 6-inch round baking pan. To assemble the rolls, place two strips of zucchini on a work surface. Spoon 2 tbsp. of ricotta mixture onto the slices and roll up. Place seam side down on top of sauce. Repeat with remaining ingredients
6. Pour remaining sauce over the rolls and sprinkle with remaining mozzarella. Cover with foil and place into the air fryer basket. Adjust the temperature to 350 Degrees F and set the timer for 20 minutes. In the last 5 minutes, remove the foil to brown the cheese. Serve immediately.
- **Nutrition Info:** Calories: 245; Protein: 15g; Fiber: 8g; Fat: 19g; Carbs: 1g

215.Korean Beef Bowl

Servings: 4
Cooking Time: 18 Minutes
Ingredients:
- 1 tablespoon minced garlic
- 1 teaspoon ground ginger
- 4 oz chive stems, chopped
- 2 tablespoon apple cider vinegar
- 1 teaspoon stevia extract
- 1 tablespoon flax seeds
- 1 teaspoon olive oil
- 1 teaspoon olive oil
- 1-pound ground beef
- 4 tablespoon chicken stock

Directions:
1. Sprinkle the ground beef with the apple cider vinegar and stir the meat with the help of the spoon.
2. After this, sprinkle the ground beef with the ground ginger, minced garlic, and olive oil.
3. Mix it up.
4. Preheat the air fryer to 370 F.
5. Put the ground beef in the air fryer basket tray and cook it for 8 minutes.
6. After this, stir the ground beef carefully and sprinkle with the chopped chives, flax seeds, olive oil, and chicken stock.
7. Mix the dish up and cook it for 10 minutes more.
8. When the time is over – stir the dish carefully.
9. Serve Korean beef bowl immediately.
10. Enjoy!

- **Nutrition Info:** calories 258, fat 10.1, fiber 1.2, carbs 4.2, protein 35.3

216.Beef Sausage With Grilled Broccoli

Servings: 4
Cooking Time: 20 Minutes
Ingredients:
- 1 pound beef Vienna sausage
- 1/2 cup mayonnaise
- 1 teaspoon yellow mustard
- 1 tablespoon fresh lemon juice
- 1 teaspoon garlic powder
- 1/4 teaspoon black pepper
- 1 pound broccoli

Directions:
1. Start by preheating your Air Fryer to 380 degrees F. Spritz the grill pan with cooking oil.
2. Cut the sausages into serving sized pieces. Cook the sausages for 15 minutes, shaking the basket occasionally to get all sides browned. Set aside.
3. In the meantime, whisk the mayonnaise with mustard, lemon juice, garlic powder, and black pepper. Toss the broccoli with the mayo mixture.
4. Turn up temperature to 400 degrees F. Cook broccoli for 6 minutes, turning halfway through the cooking time.
5. Serve the sausage with the grilled broccoli on the side.

- **Nutrition Info:** 477 Calories; 42g Fat; 3g Carbs; 19g Protein; 7g Sugars; 6g Fiber

217.Basil Tomatoes

Servings: 2
Cooking Time: 10 Minutes
Ingredients:
- 2 tomatoes, halved
- 1 tablespoon fresh basil, chopped
- Olive oil cooking spray
- Salt and black pepper, as required

Directions:
1. Preheat the Air fryer to 320 degree F and grease an Air fryer basket.
2. Spray the tomato halves evenly with olive oil cooking spray and season with salt, black pepper and basil.
3. Arrange the tomato halves into the Air fryer basket, cut sides up.
4. Cook for about 10 minutes and dish out onto serving plates.

- **Nutrition Info:** Calories: 22, Fat: 4.8g, Carbohydrates: 4.8g, Sugar: 3.2g, Protein: 1.1g, Sodium: 84mg

218.Cheesy Shrimp

Servings: 4
Cooking Time: 20 Minutes

Ingredients:
- 2/3 cup Parmesan cheese, grated
- 2 pounds shrimp, peeled and deveined
- 4 garlic cloves, minced
- 2 tablespoons olive oil
- 1 teaspoon dried basil
- ½ teaspoon dried oregano
- 1 teaspoon onion powder
- ½ teaspoon red pepper flakes, crushed
- Ground black pepper, as required
- 2 tablespoons fresh lemon juice

Directions:
1. Preheat the Air fryer to 350 degree F and grease an Air fryer basket.
2. Mix Parmesan cheese, garlic, olive oil, herbs, and spices in a large bowl.
3. Arrange half of the shrimp into the Air fryer basket in a single layer and cook for about 10 minutes.
4. Dish out the shrimps onto serving plates and drizzle with lemon juice to serve hot.
- **Nutrition Info:** Calories: 386, Fat: 14.2g, Carbohydrates: 5.3g, Sugar: 0.4g, Protein: 57.3g, Sodium: 670mg

219.Grilled Chicken Tikka Masala

Servings: 4
Cooking Time: 20 Minutes
Ingredients:
- 1 tsp. Tikka Masala 1 tsp. fine sea salt
- 2 heaping tsps. whole grain mustard
- 2 tsps. coriander, ground 2 tablespoon olive oil
- 2 large-sized chicken breasts, skinless and halved lengthwise
- 2 tsp.s onion powder
- 1½ tablespoons cider vinegar Basmati rice, steamed
- 1/3 tsp. red pepper flakes, crushed

Directions:
1. Preheat the air fryer to 335 °For 4 minutes.
2. Toss your chicken together with the other ingredients, minus basmati rice. Let it stand at least 3 hours.
3. Cook for 25 minutes in your air fryer; check for doneness because the time depending on the size of the piece of chicken.
4. Serve immediately over warm basmati rice. Enjoy!
- **Nutrition Info:** 319 Calories; 20.1g Fat; 1.9g Carbs; 30.5g Protein; 0.1g Sugars

220.Fried Spicy Tofu

Servings: 4
Cooking Time: 20 Minutes
Ingredients:
- 16 ounces firm tofu, pressed and cubed
- 1 tablespoon vegan oyster sauce
- 1 tablespoon tamari sauce
- 1 teaspoon cider vinegar
- 1 teaspoon pure maple syrup
- 1 teaspoon sriracha
- 1/2 teaspoon shallot powder
- 1/2 teaspoon porcini powder
- 1 teaspoon garlic powder
- 1 tablespoon sesame oil
- 2 tablespoons golden flaxseed meal

Directions:
1. Toss the tofu with the oyster sauce, tamari sauce, vinegar,maple syrup, sriracha, shallot powder, porcini powder, garlic powder, and sesame oil. Let it marinate for 30 minutes.
2. Toss the marinated tofu with the flaxseed meal.
3. Cook at 360 degrees F for 10 minutes; turn them over and cook for 12 minutes more.
- **Nutrition Info:** 173 Calories; 13g Fat; 5g Carbs; 12g Protein; 8g Sugars; 1g Fiber

221.Indian Meatballs With Lamb

Servings: 8
Cooking Time: 14 Minutes
Ingredients:
- 1 garlic clove
- 1 tablespoon butter
- 4 oz chive stems
- ¼ tablespoon turmeric
- 1/3 teaspoon cayenne pepper
- 1 teaspoon ground coriander
- ¼ teaspoon bay leaf
- 1 teaspoon salt
- 1-pound ground lamb
- 1 egg
- 1 teaspoon ground black pepper

Directions:
1. Peel the garlic clove and mince it
2. Combine the minced garlic with the ground lamb.
3. Then sprinkle the meat mixture with the turmeric, cayenne pepper, ground coriander, bay leaf, salt, and ground black pepper.
4. Beat the egg in the forcemeat.
5. Then grate the chives and add them in the lamb forcemeat too.
6. Mix it up to make the smooth mass.
7. Then preheat the air fryer to 400 F.
8. Put the butter in the air fryer basket tray and melt it.
9. Then make the meatballs from the lamb mixture and place them in the air fryer basket tray.
10. Cook the dish for 14 minutes.
11. Stir the meatballs twice during the cooking.
12. Serve the cooked meatballs immediately.
13. Enjoy!
- **Nutrition Info:** calories 134, fat 6.2, fiber 0.4, carbs 1.8, protein 16.9

222. Creamy Breaded Shrimp

Servings: 3
Cooking Time: 20 Minutes
Ingredients:
- ¼ cup all-purpose flour
- 1 cup panko breadcrumbs
- 1 pound shrimp, peeled and deveined
- ½ cup mayonnaise
- ¼ cup sweet chili sauce
- 1 tablespoon Sriracha sauce

Directions:
1. Preheat the Air fryer to 400-degree F and grease an Air fryer basket.
2. Place flour in a shallow bowl and mix the mayonnaise, chili sauce, and Sriracha sauce in another bowl.
3. Place the breadcrumbs in a third bowl.
4. Coat each shrimp with the flour, dip into mayonnaise mixture and finally, dredge in the breadcrumbs.
5. Arrange half of the coated shrimps into the Air fryer basket and cook for about 10 minutes.
6. Dish out the coated shrimps onto serving plates and repeat with the remaining mixture.
- **Nutrition Info:** Calories: 540, Fat: 18.2g, Carbohydrates: 33.1g, Sugar: 10.6g, Protein: 36.8g, Sodium: 813mg

223. Vegetable Cane

Servings: 4
Cooking Time: More Than 60 Minutes;
Ingredients:
- 2 calf legs
- 4 carrots
- 4 medium potatoes
- 1 clove garlic
- 300ml Broth
- Leave to taste
- Pepper to taste

Directions:
1. Place the ears, garlic, and half of the broth in the greased basket.
2. Set the temperature to 1800C.
3. Cook the stems for 40 minutes, turning them in the middle of cooking.
4. Add the vegetables in pieces, salt, pepper, pour the rest of the broth and cook for another 50 minutes (time may vary depending on the size of the hocks).
5. Mix the vegetables and the ears 2 to 3 times during cooking.
- **Nutrition Info:** Calories 7.9, Fat 0.49g, Carbohydrate 0.77g, Sugar 0.49g, Protein 0.08mg, Cholesterol 0mg

224. Christmas Filet Mignon Steak

Servings: 6
Cooking Time: 20 Minutes

Ingredients:
- 1/3 stick butter, at room temperature
- 1/2 cup heavy cream
- 1/2 medium-sized garlic bulb, peeled and pressed
- 6 filet mignon steaks
- 2 teaspoons mixed peppercorns, freshly cracked
- 1 ½ tablespoons apple cider
- A dash of hot sauce
- 1 ½ teaspoons sea salt flakes

Directions:
1. Season the mignon steaks with the cracked peppercorns and salt flakes. Roast the mignon steaks in the preheated Air Fryer for 24 minutes at 385 degrees F, turning once. Check for doneness and set aside, keeping it warm.
2. In a small nonstick saucepan that is placed over a moderate flame, mash the garlic to a smooth paste. Whisk in the rest of the above ingredients. Whisk constantly until it has a uniform consistency.
3. To finish, lay the filet mignon steaks on serving plates; spoon a little sauce onto each filet mignon.
- **Nutrition Info:** 452 Calories; 32g Fat; 8g Carbs; 26g Protein; 6g Sugars; 1g Fiber

225. Steak With Cascabel-garlic Sauce

Servings: 4
Cooking Time: 20 Minutes
Ingredients:
- 2 teaspoons brown mustard
- 2 tablespoons mayonnaise
- 1 ½ pounds beef flank steak, trimmed and cubed
- 2 teaspoons minced cascabel
- ½ cup scallions, finely chopped
- 1/3 cup Crème fraîche
- 2 teaspoons cumin seeds
- 3 cloves garlic, pressed
- Pink peppercorns to taste, freshly cracked
- 1 teaspoon fine table salt
- 1/3 teaspoon black pepper, preferably freshly ground

Directions:
1. Firstly, fry the cumin seeds just about 1 minute or until they pop.
2. After that, season your beef flank steak with fine table salt, black pepper and the fried cumin seeds; arrange the seasoned beef cubes on the bottom of your baking dish that fits in the air fryer.
3. Throw in the minced cascabel, garlic, and scallions; air-fry approximately 8 minutes at 390 degrees F.
4. Once the beef cubes start to tender, add your favorite mayo, Crème fraîche, freshly cracked pink peppercorns and mustard; air-

fry 7 minutes longer. Serve over hot wild rice.

- **Nutrition Info:** 329 Calories; 16g Fat; 8g Carbs; 37g Protein; 9g Sugars; 6g Fiber

226.Lobster Lasagna Maine Style

Servings: 6
Cooking Time: 50 Minutes
Ingredients:
- 1/2 (15 ounces) container ricotta cheese
- 1 egg
- 1 cup shredded Cheddar cheese
- 1/2 cup shredded mozzarella cheese
- 1/2 cup grated Parmesan cheese
- 1/2 medium onion, minced
- 1-1/2 teaspoons minced garlic
- 1 tablespoon chopped fresh parsley
- 1/2 teaspoon freshly ground black pepper
- 1 (16 ounces) jar Alfredo pasta sauce
- 8 no-boil lasagna noodles
- 1 pound cooked and cubed lobster meat
- 5-ounce package baby spinach leaves

Directions:
1. Mix well half of Parmesan, half of the mozzarella, half of cheddar, egg, and ricotta cheese in a medium bowl. Stir in pepper, parsley, garlic, and onion.
2. Place the instant pot air fryer lid on, lightly grease baking pan of the instant pot with cooking spray.
3. On the bottom of the pan, spread ½ of the Alfredo sauce, top with a single layer of lasagna noodles. Followed by 1/3 of lobster meat, 1/3 of ricotta cheese mixture, 1/3 of spinach. Repeat layering process until all ingredients are used up.
4. Sprinkle remaining cheese on top. Shake pan to settle lasagna and burst bubbles. Cover pan with foil and place the baking pan in the instant pot.
5. Close the air fryer lid and cook at 360 ºF for 30 minutes
6. Remove foil and cook for 10 minutes at 390 ºF until tops are lightly browned.
7. Let it stand for 10 minutes.
8. Serve and enjoy.
- **Nutrition Info:** Calories: 558; Carbs: 20.4g; Protein: 36.8g; Fat: 36.5g

227.Coco Mug Cake

Servings: 1
Cooking Time: 20 Minutes
Ingredients:
- 1 large egg.
- 2 tbsp. granular erythritol.
- 2 tbsp. coconut flour.
- 2 tbsp. heavy whipping cream.

- ¼ tsp. baking powder.
- ¼ tsp. vanilla extract.

Directions:
1. In a 4-inch ramekin, whisk egg, then add remaining ingredients. Stir until smooth. Place into the air fryer basket.
2. Adjust the temperature to 300 Degrees F and set the timer for 25 minutes.
3. When done a toothpick should come out clean. Enjoy right out of the ramekin with a spoon. Serve warm.
- **Nutrition Info:** Calories: 237; Protein: 9g; Fiber: 0g; Fat: 14g; Carbs: 47g

228.Coconut-crusted Haddock With Curried Pumpkin Seeds

Servings: 4
Cooking Time: 10 Minutes
Ingredients:
- 2 teaspoons canola oil
- 2 teaspoons honey
- 1 teaspoon curry powder
- 1/4 teaspoon ground cinnamon
- 1 teaspoon salt
- 1 cup pumpkin seeds
- 1-1/2 pounds haddock or cod filets
- 1/2 cup roughly grated unsweetened coconut
- 3/4 cups panko-style bread crumbs
- 2 tablespoons butter, melted
- 3 tablespoons apricot fruit spread
- 1 tablespoon lime juice

Directions:
1. Start by preheating toaster oven to 350°F.
2. In a medium bowl, mix honey, oil, curry powder, 1/2 teaspoon salt, and cinnamon.
3. Add pumpkin seeds to the bowl and toss to coat, then lay flat on a baking sheet.
4. Toast for 14 minutes, then transfer to a bowl to cool.
5. Increase the oven temperature to 450°F.
6. Brush a baking sheet with oil and lay filets flat.
7. In another medium mixing bowl, mix together bread crumbs, butter, and remaining salt.
8. In a small bowl mash together apricot spread and lime juice.
9. Brush each filet with apricot mixture, then press bread crumb mixture onto each piece.
10. Bake for 10 minutes.
11. Transfer to a plate and top with pumpkin seeds to serve.
- **Nutrition Info:** Calories: 273, Sodium: 491 mg, Dietary Fiber: 6.1 g, Total Fat: 8.4 g, Total Carbs: 47.3 g, Protein: 7.0 g.

MEAT RECIPES

229.Simple Herbed Hens

Servings:8
Cooking Time: 30 Minutes
Ingredients:
- 4 (1¼-pound / 567-g) Cornish hens, giblets removed, split lengthwise
- 2 cups white wine, divided
- 2 garlic cloves, minced
- 1 small onion, minced
- ½ teaspoon celery seeds
- ½ teaspoon poultry seasoning
- ½ teaspoon paprika
- ½ teaspoon dried oregano
- ¼ teaspoon freshly ground black pepper

Directions:
1. Place the hens, cavity side up, in the baking pan. Pour 1½ cups of the wine over the hens. Set aside.
2. In a shallow bowl, combine the garlic, onion, celery seeds, poultry seasoning, paprika, oregano, and pepper. Sprinkle half of the combined seasonings over the cavity of each split half. Cover and refrigerate. Allow the hens to marinate for 2 hours.
3. Transfer the hens to the pan. Slide the baking pan into Rack Position 1, select Convection Bake, set temperature to 350ºF (180ºC) and set time to 90 minutes.
4. Flip the breast halfway through and remove the skin. Pour the remaining ½ cup of wine over the top, and sprinkle with the remaining seasonings.
5. When cooking is complete, the inner temperature of the hens should be at least 165ºF (74ºC). Transfer the hens to a serving platter and serve hot.

230.Chicken With Potatoes And Corn

Servings:4
Cooking Time: 25 Minutes
Ingredients:
- 4 bone-in, skin-on chicken thighs
- 2 teaspoons kosher salt, divided
- 1 cup Bisquick baking mix
- ½ cup butter, melted, divided
- 1 pound (454 g) small red potatoes, quartered
- 3 ears corn, shucked and cut into rounds 1- to 1½-inches thick
- $1/3$ cup heavy whipping cream
- ½ teaspoon freshly ground black pepper

Directions:
1. Sprinkle the chicken on all sides with 1 teaspoon of kosher salt. Place the baking mix in a shallow dish. Brush the thighs on all sides with ¼ cup of butter, then dredge them in the baking mix, coating them all on

sides. Place the chicken in the center of the baking pan.
2. Place the potatoes in a large bowl with 2 tablespoons of butter and toss to coat. Place them on one side of the chicken on the pan.
3. Place the corn in a medium bowl and drizzle with the remaining butter. Sprinkle with ¼ teaspoon of kosher salt and toss to coat. Place on the pan on the other side of the chicken.
4. Slide the baking pan into Rack Position 2, select Roast, set temperature to 375ºF (190ºC), and set time to 25 minutes.
5. After 20 minutes, remove from the oven and put the potatoes back to the bowl. Return the pan to oven and continue cooking.
6. As the chicken continues cooking, add the cream, black pepper, and remaining kosher salt to the potatoes. Lightly mash the potatoes with a potato masher.
7. When cooking is complete, the corn should be tender and the chicken cooked through, reading 165ºF (74ºC) on a meat thermometer. Remove from the oven. Serve the chicken with the smashed potatoes and corn on the side.

231.Cheesy Chicken With Tomato Sauce

Servings:2
Cooking Time: 20 Minutes
Ingredients:
- 2 chicken breasts, ½-inch thick
- 1 egg, beaten
- ½ cup breadcrumbs
- Salt and black pepper to taste
- 2 tbsp tomato sauce
- 2 tbsp Grana Padano cheese, grated
- ¼ cup mozzarella cheese, shredded

Directions:
1. Preheat on AirFry function to 350 F. Dip the breasts into the egg, then into the crumbs and arrange on the greased basket. Cook for 5 minutes. Turn, drizzle with tomato sauce, sprinkle with Grana Padano and mozzarella cheeses, and cook for 5 more minutes. Serve warm.

232.Garlic-buttery Chicken Wings

Servings: 4
Cooking Time: 20 Minutes
Ingredients:
- 12 chicken wings
- ¼ cup butter
- ¼ cup honey
- ½ tbsp salt
- 4 garlic cloves, minced
- ¾ cup potato starch

Directions:

1. Preheat on Air Fry function to 370 F. Coat chicken with potato starch. Transfer to the greased Air Fryer basket and fit in the baking tray. Cook for 5 minutes. Whisk the rest of the ingredients in a bowl. Pour the sauce over the wings and serve.

233.Crispy Crusted Chicken

Servings: 4
Cooking Time: 30 Minutes
Ingredients:

- 4 chicken breasts, skinless and boneless
- 2 tbsp butter, melted
- 3 cups corn flakes, crushed
- 1 tsp poultry seasoning
- 1 tsp water
- 1 egg, lightly beaten
- Pepper
- Salt

Directions:

1. Fit the oven with the rack in position
2. Season chicken with poultry seasoning, pepper, and salt.
3. In a shallow dish, whisk together egg and water.
4. In a separate shallow dish, mix crushed cornflakes and melted butter.
5. Dip chicken into the egg mixture then coats with crushed cornflakes.
6. Place the coated chicken into the parchment-lined baking pan.
7. Set to bake at 400 F for 35 minutes. After 5 minutes place the baking pan in the preheated oven.
8. Serve and enjoy.
- **Nutrition Info:** Calories 421 Fat 17.7 g Carbohydrates 18.6 g Sugar 1.5 g Protein 45.1 g Cholesterol 186 mg

234.Bacon Wrapped Pork Tenderloin

Servings: 4
Cooking Time: 15 Minutes
Ingredients:

- Pork:
- 1-2 tbsp. Dijon mustard
- 3-4 strips of bacon
- 1 pork tenderloin
- Apple Gravy:
- ½ - 1 tsp. Dijon mustard
- 1 tbsp. almond flour
- 2 tbsp. ghee
- 1 chopped onion
- 2-3 Granny Smith apples
- 1 C. vegetable broth

Directions:

1. Preparing the Ingredients. Spread Dijon mustard all over tenderloin and wrap the meat with strips of bacon.

2. Air Frying. Place into the air fryer oven, set temperature to 360°F, and set time to 15 minutes and cook 10-15 minutes at 360 degrees. Use a meat thermometer to check for doneness.
3. To make sauce, heat ghee in a pan and add shallots. Cook 1-2 minutes.
4. Then add apples, cooking 3-5 minutes until softened.
5. Add flour and ghee to make a roux. Add broth and mustard, stirring well to combine.
6. When the sauce starts to bubble, add 1 cup of sautéed apples, cooking till sauce thickens.
7. Once pork tenderloin I cook, allow to sit 5-10 minutes to rest before slicing.
8. Serve topped with apple gravy.
- **Nutrition Info:** CALORIES: 552; FAT: 25G; PROTEIN:29G; SUGAR:6G

235.Spicy Pork Lettuce Wraps

Servings:4
Cooking Time: 12 Minutes
Ingredients:

- 1 (1-pound / 454-g) medium pork tenderloin, silver skin and external fat trimmed
- $^2/_3$ cup soy sauce, divided
- 1 teaspoon cornstarch
- 1 medium jalapeño, deseeded and minced
- 1 can diced water chestnuts
- ½ large red bell pepper, deseeded and chopped
- 2 scallions, chopped, white and green parts separated
- 1 head butter lettuce
- ½ cup roasted, chopped almonds
- ¼ cup coarsely chopped cilantro

Directions:

1. Cut the tenderloin into ¼-inch slices and place them in the baking pan. Baste with about 3 tablespoons of soy sauce. Stir the cornstarch into the remaining sauce and set aside.
2. Slide the baking pan into Rack Position 2, select Roast, set temperature to 375ºF (190ºC), and set time to 12 minutes.
3. After 5 minutes, remove from the oven. Place the pork slices on a cutting board. Place the jalapeño, water chestnuts, red pepper, and the white parts of the scallions in the baking pan and pour the remaining sauce over. Stir to coat the vegetables with the sauce. Return the pan to the oven and continue cooking.
4. While the vegetables cook, chop the pork into small pieces. Separate the lettuce leaves, discarding any tough outer leaves and setting aside the small inner leaves for

another use. You'll want 12 to 18 leaves, depending on size and your appetites.

5. After 5 minutes, remove from the oven. Add the pork to the vegetables, stirring to combine. Return the pan to the oven and continue cooking for the remaining 2 minutes until the pork is warmed back up and the sauce has reduced slightly.

6. When cooking is complete, remove from the oven. Place the pork and vegetables in a medium serving bowl and stir in half the green parts of the scallions. To serve, spoon some pork and vegetables into each of the lettuce leaves. Top with the remaining scallion greens and garnish with the nuts and cilantro.

236.Air Fried Chicken Wings With Buffalo Sauce

Servings:6
Cooking Time: 20 Minutes
Ingredients:
- 16 chicken drumettes (party wings)
- Chicken seasoning or rub, to taste
- 1 teaspoon garlic powder
- Ground black pepper, to taste
- ¼ cup buffalo wings sauce
- Cooking spray

Directions:
1. Spritz the air fryer basket with cooking spray.
2. Rub the chicken wings with chicken seasoning, garlic powder, and ground black pepper on a clean work surface.
3. Arrange the chicken wings in the basket. Spritz with cooking spray.
4. Put the air fryer basket on the baking pan and slide into Rack Position 2, select Air Fry, set temperature to 400ºF (205ºC) and set time to 10 minutes.
5. Flip the chicken wings halfway through.
6. When cooking is complete, the chicken wings should be lightly browned.
7. Transfer the chicken wings in a large bowl, then pour in the buffalo wings sauce and toss to coat well.
8. Put the wings back to the oven and set time to 7 minutes. Flip the wings halfway through.
9. When cooking is complete, the wings should be heated through. Serve immediately.

237.Tender Pork Tenderloin

Servings: 4
Cooking Time: 20 Minutes
Ingredients:
- 1 1/2 lbs pork tenderloin
- 1 tsp garlic powder
- 1 tsp Italian seasoning

- 2 tbsp olive oil
- 1 tsp ground coriander
- 1/4 tsp pepper
- 1 tsp sea salt

Directions:
1. Fit the oven with the rack in position
2. Brush pork tenderloin with 1 tablespoon of olive oil.
3. Mix coriander, garlic powder, Italian seasoning, pepper, and salt and rub over pork tenderloin.
4. Heat remaining oil in a pan over medium-high heat.
5. Add pork tenderloin in a pan and sear until brown.
6. Place pork tenderloin in baking pan.
7. Set to bake at 400 F for 25 minutes. After 5 minutes place the baking pan in the preheated oven.
8. Slice and serve.
- **Nutrition Info:** Calories 310 Fat 13.3 g Carbohydrates 0.7 g Sugar 0.3 g Protein 44.7 g Cholesterol 125 mg

238.Air Fry Chicken Drumsticks

Servings: 6
Cooking Time: 25 Minutes
Ingredients:
- 6 chicken drumsticks
- 1/2 tsp garlic powder
- 2 tbsp olive oil
- 1/2 tsp ground cumin
- 3/4 tsp paprika
- Pepper
- Salt

Directions:
1. Fit the oven with the rack in position 2.
2. Add chicken drumsticks and olive oil in a large bowl and toss well.
3. Sprinkle garlic powder, paprika, cumin, pepper, and salt over chicken drumsticks and toss until well coated.
4. Place chicken drumsticks in the air fryer basket then place an air fryer basket in the baking pan.
5. Place a baking pan on the oven rack. Set to air fry at 400 F for 25 minutes.
6. Serve and enjoy.
- **Nutrition Info:** Calories 120 Fat 7.4 g Carbohydrates 0.4 g Sugar 0.1 g Protein 12.8 g Cholesterol 40 mg

239.Sweet Pork Meatballs With Cheddar Cheese

Servings:4
Cooking Time: 25 Minutes
Ingredients:
- 1 lb ground pork
- 1 large onion, chopped

- ½ tsp maple syrup
- 2 tsp yellow mustard
- ½ cup fresh basil leaves, chopped
- Salt and black pepper to taste
- 2 tbsp Cheddar cheese, grated

Directions:

1. In a bowl, add ground pork, onion, maple syrup, mustard, basil, salt, pepper, and cheddar cheese; mix well. Form balls. Place in the frying basket. Select AirFry function, adjust the temperature to 400 F, and press Start. Cook for 10 minutes, shake, and cook for 5 minutes.

240.Baked Sweet & Tangy Pork Chops

Servings: 2
Cooking Time: 35 Minutes
Ingredients:

- 2 pork chops
- 2 tbsp brown sugar
- 2 tbsp ketchup
- 2 onion sliced
- Pepper
- Salt

Directions:

1. Fit the oven with the rack in position
2. Season pork chops with pepper and salt.
3. Place pork chops in a baking dish.
4. Mix ketchup and brown sugar and pour over pork chops.
5. Top with onion slices.
6. Set to bake at 375 F for 40 minutes. After 5 minutes place the baking dish in the preheated oven.
7. Serve and enjoy.

- **Nutrition Info:** Calories 308 Fat 19.9 g Carbohydrates 13.5 g Sugar 12.5 g Protein 18.4 g Cholesterol 69 mg

241.Golden Lamb Chops

Servings:4
Cooking Time: 25 Minutes
Ingredients:

- 1 cup all-purpose flour
- 2 teaspoons dried sage leaves
- 2 teaspoons garlic powder
- 1 tablespoon mild paprika
- 1 tablespoon salt
- 4 (6-ounce / 170-g) bone-in lamb shoulder chops, fat trimmed
- Cooking spray

Directions:

1. Spritz the air fryer basket with cooking spray.
2. Combine the flour, sage leaves, garlic powder, paprika, and salt in a large bowl. Stir to mix well. Dunk in the lamb chops and toss to coat well.

3. Arrange the lamb chops in the pan and spritz with cooking spray.
4. Put the air fryer basket on the baking pan and slide into Rack Position 2, select Air Fry, set temperature to 375ºF (190ºC) and set time to 25 minutes.
5. Flip the chops halfway through.
6. When cooking is complete, the chops should be golden brown and reaches your desired doneness.
7. Serve immediately.

242.Tuscan Air Fried Veal Loin

Servings: 3 Veal Chops
Cooking Time: 12 Minutes
Ingredients:

- 1½ teaspoons crushed fennel seeds
- 1 tablespoon minced fresh rosemary leaves
- 1 tablespoon minced garlic
- 1½ teaspoons lemon zest
- 1½ teaspoons salt
- ½ teaspoon red pepper flakes
- 2 tablespoons olive oil
- 3 (10-ounce / 284-g) bone-in veal loin, about ½ inch thick

Directions:

1. Combine all the ingredients, except for the veal loin, in a large bowl. Stir to mix well.
2. Dunk the loin in the mixture and press to submerge. Wrap the bowl in plastic and refrigerate for at least an hour to marinate.
3. Arrange the veal loin in the basket.
4. Put the air fryer basket on the baking pan and slide into Rack Position 2, select Air Fry, set temperature to 400ºF (205ºC) and set time to 12 minutes.
5. Flip the veal halfway through.
6. When cooking is complete, the internal temperature of the veal should reach at least 145ºF (63ºC) for medium rare.
7. Serve immediately.

243.Copycat Taco Bell Crunch Wraps

Servings: 6
Cooking Time: 2 Minutes
Ingredients:

- 6 wheat tostadas
- 2 C. sour cream
- 2 C. Mexican blend cheese
- 2 C. shredded lettuce
- 12 ounces low-sodium nacho cheese
- 3 Roma tomatoes
- 6 12-inch wheat tortillas
- 1 1/3 C. water
- 2 packets low-sodium taco seasoning
- 2 pounds of lean ground beef

Directions:

1. Preparing the Ingredients. Ensure your air fryer oven is preheated to 400 degrees.

2. Make beef according to taco seasoning packets.
3. Place 2/3 C. prepared beef, 4 tbsp. cheese, 1 tostada, 1/3 C. sour cream, 1/3 C. lettuce, 1/6th of tomatoes and 1/3 C. cheese on each tortilla.
4. Fold up tortillas edges and repeat with remaining ingredients.
5. Lay the folded sides of tortillas down into the air fryer oven and spray with olive oil.
6. Air Frying. Set temperature to 400°F, and set time to 2 minutes. Cook 2 minutes till browned.
- **Nutrition Info:** CALORIES: 311; FAT: 9G; PROTEIN:22G; SUGAR:2

244.Bacon-wrapped Chicken Breasts

Servings:2
Cooking Time: 20 Minutes
Ingredients:
- 2 chicken breasts
- 8 oz onion and chive cream cheese
- 1 tbsp butter
- 6 turkey bacon
- Salt to taste
- 1 tbsp fresh parsley, chopped
- Juice from ½ lemon

Directions:
1. Preheat on AirFry function to 390 F. Stretch out the bacon slightly and lay them in 2 sets; 3 bacon strips together on each side. Place the chicken breast on each bacon set and use a knife to smear cream cheese on both.
2. Share the butter on top and sprinkle with salt. Wrap the bacon around the chicken and secure the ends into the wrap. Place the wrapped chicken in the basket and press Start.
3. Cook for 14 minutes. Remove the chicken onto a serving platter and top with parsley and lemon juice. Serve with steamed greens.

245.Gnocchi With Chicken And Spinach

Servings:4
Cooking Time: 13 Minutes
Ingredients:
- 1 (1-pound / 454-g) package shelf-stable gnocchi
- 1¼ cups chicken stock
- ½ teaspoon kosher salt
- 1 pound (454 g) chicken breast, cut into 1-inch chunks
- 1 cup heavy whipping cream
- 2 tablespoons sun-dried tomato purée
- 1 garlic clove, minced
- 1 cup frozen spinach, thawed and drained
- 1 cup grated Parmesan cheese

Directions:

1. Place the gnocchi in an even layer in the baking pan. Pour the chicken stock over the gnocchi.
2. Slide the baking pan into Rack Position 1, select Convection Bake, set temperature to 450ºF (235ºC), and set time to 7 minutes.
3. While the gnocchi are cooking, sprinkle the salt over the chicken pieces. In a small bowl, mix the cream, tomato purée, and garlic.
4. When cooking is complete, blot off any remaining stock, or drain the gnocchi and return it to the pan. Top the gnocchi with the spinach and chicken. Pour the cream mixture over the ingredients in the pan.
5. Slide the baking pan into Rack Position 2, select Roast, set temperature to 400ºF (205ºC), and set time to 6 minutes.
6. After 4 minutes, remove from the oven and gently stir the ingredients. Return to the oven and continue cooking.
7. When cooking is complete, the gnocchi should be tender and the chicken should be cooked through. Remove from the oven. Stir in the Parmesan cheese until it's melted and serve.

246.Cheesy Chicken In Leek-tomato Sauce

Servings: 4
Cooking Time: 20 Minutes
Ingredients:
- 2 large-sized chicken breasts, cut in half lengthwise
- Salt and ground black pepper, to taste
- 4 ounces Cheddar cheese, cut into sticks
- 1 tablespoon sesame oil
- 1 cup leeks, chopped
- 2 cloves garlic, minced
- 2/3 cup roasted vegetable stock
- 2/3 cup tomato puree
- 1 teaspoon dried rosemary
- 1 teaspoon dried thyme

Directions:
1. Preparing the Ingredients. Firstly, season chicken breasts with the salt and black pepper; place a piece of Cheddar cheese in the middle. Then, tie it using a kitchen string; drizzle with sesame oil and reserve.
2. Add the leeks and garlic to the oven safe bowl.
3. Air Frying. Cook in the air fryer oven at 390 degrees F for 5 minutes or until tender.
4. Add the reserved chicken. Throw in the other ingredients and cook for 12 to 13 minutes more or until the chicken is done. Enjoy!

247.Flavorful Sirloin Steak

Servings: 2
Cooking Time: 14 Minutes
Ingredients:

- 1 lb sirloin steaks
- 1/2 tsp garlic powder
- 1/2 tsp onion powder
- 1/4 tsp smoked paprika
- 1 tsp olive oil
- Pepper
- Salt

Directions:
1. Fit the oven with the rack in position 2.
2. Line the air fryer basket with parchment paper.
3. Brush steak with olive oil and rub with garlic powder, onion powder, paprika, pepper, and salt.
4. Place the steak in the air fryer basket then places an air fryer basket in the baking pan.
5. Place a baking pan on the oven rack. Set to air fry at 400 F for 14 minutes.
6. Serve and enjoy.
- **Nutrition Info:** Calories 447 Fat 16.5 g Carbohydrates 1.2 g Sugar 0.4 g Protein 69 g Cholesterol 203 mg

248.Crispy Crusted Pork Chops

Servings: 2
Cooking Time: 15 Minutes
Ingredients:
- 2 pork chops, bone-in
- 1 cup pork rinds, crushed
- 1/2 tsp parsley
- 1 tbsp olive oil
- 1/2 tsp garlic powder
- 1/2 tsp onion powder
- 1/2 tsp paprika

Directions:
1. Fit the oven with the rack in position 2.
2. In a large bowl, mix pork rinds, garlic powder, onion powder, parsley, and paprika.
3. Brush pork chops with oil and coat with pork rind mixture.
4. place coated pork chops in air fryer basket then place air fryer basket in baking pan.
5. Place a baking pan on the oven rack. Set to air fry at 400 F for 15 minutes.
6. Serve and enjoy.
- **Nutrition Info:** Calories 413 Fat 32.7 g Carbohydrates 1.3 g Sugar 0.4 g Protein 28.5 g Cholesterol 92 mg

249.Baked Italian Lemon Chicken

Servings: 4
Cooking Time: 25 Minutes
Ingredients:
- 1 1/4 lbs chicken breasts, skinless and boneless
- 3 tbsp butter, melted
- 1 tsp Italian seasoning
- 1 tbsp olive oil
- 1 tbsp fresh parsley, chopped

- 2 tbsp fresh lemon juice
- 1/4 cup water
- Pepper
- Salt

Directions:
1. Fit the oven with the rack in position
2. Season chicken with Italian seasoning, pepper, and salt.
3. Heat oil in a pan over medium-high heat.
4. Add chicken to the pan and cook for 3-5 minutes on each side.
5. Transfer chicken to a baking dish.
6. In a small bowl, mix together butter, lemon juice, and water.
7. Pour butter mixture over chicken.
8. Set to bake at 400 F for 30 minutes. After 5 minutes place the baking dish in the preheated oven.
9. Garnish with parsley and serve.
- **Nutrition Info:** Calories 382 Fat 23.1 g Carbohydrates 0.4 g Sugar 0.3 g Protein 41.2 g Cholesterol 150 mg

250.Shrimp Paste Chicken

Servings: 2
Cooking Time: 30 Minutes
Ingredients:
- 6 chicken wings
- ½ tbsp sugar
- 2 tbsp cornflour
- 1 tbsp white wine
- 1 tbsp shrimp paste
- 1 tbsp grated ginger
- ½ tbsp olive oil

Directions:
1. In a bowl, mix shrimp paste, olive oil, ginger, white wine, and sugar. Cover the chicken wings with the prepared marinade and roll in the flour.
2. Place the chicken in the greased baking dish and cook in your for 20 minutes at 350 F on Air Fry function. Serve.

251.Lemon Mustard Chicken

Servings: 4
Cooking Time: 20 Minutes
Ingredients:
- 1 lbs chicken tenders
- 1 garlic clove, minced
- 1/2 oz fresh lemon juice
- 1/2 tsp pepper
- 2 tbsp fresh tarragon, chopped
- 1/2 cup whole grain mustard
- 1/2 tsp paprika
- 1/4 tsp kosher salt

Directions:
1. Fit the oven with the rack in position
2. Add all ingredients except chicken to the large bowl and mix well.

3. Add chicken to the bowl and stir until well coated.
4. Place chicken in a baking dish.
5. Set to bake at 425 F for 25 minutes. After 5 minutes place the baking dish in the preheated oven.
6. Serve and enjoy.
- **Nutrition Info:** Calories 242 Fat 9.5 g Carbohydrates 3.1 g Sugar 0.1 g Protein 33.2 g Cholesterol 101 mg

252.Lechon Kawali

Servings:4
Cooking Time: 30 Minutes
Ingredients:
- 1 pound (454 g) pork belly, cut into three thick chunks
- 6 garlic cloves
- 2 bay leaves
- 2 tablespoons soy sauce
- 1 teaspoon kosher salt
- 1 teaspoon ground black pepper
- 3 cups water
- Cooking spray

Directions:
1. Put all the ingredients in a pressure cooker, then put the lid on and cook on high for 15 minutes.
2. Natural release the pressure and release any remaining pressure, transfer the tender pork belly on a clean work surface. Allow to cool under room temperature until you can handle.
3. Generously Spritz the air fryer basket with cooking spray.
4. Cut each chunk into two slices, then put the pork slices in the pan.
5. Put the air fryer basket on the baking pan and slide into Rack Position 2, select Air Fry, set temperature to 400ºF (205ºC) and set time to 15 minutes.
6. After 7 minutes, remove from the oven. Flip the pork. Return to the oven and continue cooking.
7. When cooking is complete, the pork fat should be crispy.
8. Serve immediately.

253.Potato Garlic Chicken

Servings: 4
Cooking Time: 25 Minutes
Ingredients:
- 4 chicken breasts, skinless & boneless
- 1/2 cup cheddar cheese, shredded
- 1 cup mozzarella cheese, shredded
- 2 tsp dried parsley
- 1/2 tsp crushed red pepper
- 1 tbsp garlic, minced
- 1/2 cup butter

- 1 lb baby potatoes, cut into half
- 1/4 tsp pepper
- 1/4 tsp salt

Directions:
1. Fit the oven with the rack in position
2. Season chicken with pepper and salt and place in a casserole dish. Top with potatoes.
3. Melt butter in a pan over medium heat. Add garlic and sauté for a minute.
4. Remove pan from heat and let it cool for 5 minutes.
5. Pour melted butter over chicken and potatoes. Sprinkle with pepper and parsley.
6. Set to bake at 400 F for 25 minutes. After 5 minutes place the casserole dish in the preheated oven.
7. Remove the casserole dish from the oven. Sprinkle mozzarella cheese and cheddar cheese on top of chicken and potatoes and bake for 5 minutes more.
8. Serve and enjoy.
- **Nutrition Info:** Calories 635 Fat 40 g Carbohydrates 16.8 g Sugar 0.3 g Protein 51.6 g Cholesterol 210 mg

254.Ham And Eggs

Servings:x
Cooking Time:x
Ingredients:
- Bread slices (brown or white)
- 1 egg white for every 2 slices
- 1 tsp sugar for every 2 slices
- ½ lb. sliced ham

Directions:
1. Put two slices together and cut them along the diagonal. In a bowl, whisk the egg whites and add some sugar.
2. Dip the bread triangles into this mixture. Cook the chicken now. Pre heat the oven at 180° C for 4 minutes. Place the coated bread triangles in the fry basket and close it. Let them cook at the same temperature for another 20 minutes at least.
3. Halfway through the process, turn the triangles over so that you get a uniform cook. Top with ham and serve.

255.Juicy Chicken Patties

Servings: 4
Cooking Time: 25 Minutes
Ingredients:
- 1 egg
- 1 lb ground chicken
- 1 tsp garlic, minced
- 1/2 cup onion, minced
- 3/4 cup breadcrumbs
- 1/2 cup mozzarella cheese, grated cheese
- 1 cup carrot, grated
- 1 cup cauliflower, grated

- 1/8 tsp pepper
- 3/4 tsp salt

Directions:
1. Fit the oven with the rack in position
2. Add all ingredients into the mixing bowl and mix until well combined.
3. Make 4 equal shapes of patties from meat mixture and place onto the parchment-lined baking pan.
4. Set to bake at 400 F for 30 minutes. After 5 minutes place the baking pan in the preheated oven.
5. Serve and enjoy.
- **Nutrition Info:** Calories 346 Fat 11.2 g Carbohydrates 20.4 g Sugar 3.9 g Protein 38.8 g Cholesterol 144 mg

256.Air Fryer Chicken Tenders

Servings: 4
Cooking Time: 16 Minutes
Ingredients:
- 1 lb chicken tenders
- For rub:
- 1/2 tbsp dried thyme
- 1 tbsp garlic powder
- 1 tbsp paprika
- 1/2 tbsp onion powder
- 1/2 tsp cayenne pepper
- Pepper
- Salt

Directions:
1. Fit the oven with the rack in position 2.
2. In a bowl, add all rub ingredients and mix well.
3. Add chicken tenders into the bowl and coat well.
4. Place chicken tenders in the air fryer basket then place an air fryer basket in the baking pan.
5. Place a baking pan on the oven rack. Set to air fry at 370 F for 16 minutes.
6. Serve and enjoy.
- **Nutrition Info:** Calories 232 Fat 8.7 g Carbohydrates 3.6 g Sugar 1 g Protein 33.6 g Cholesterol 101 mg

257.Stuffed Bell Peppers

Servings: 6
Cooking Time: 15 Minutes
Ingredients:
- 6 green bell peppers, cut off tops & remove seeds
- 1 lb. lean ground beef
- 1 tbsp. olive oil
- ¼ cup green onion, chopped
- ¼ cup fresh parsley, chopped
- ½ tsp sage
- ½ tsp garlic salt
- 1 cup rice, cooked

- 1 cup marinara sauce
- Nonstick cooking spray
- ¼ cup mozzarella cheese, grated

Directions:
1. Heat a medium skillet over med-high heat. Add ground beef and cook, breaking up with spatula, until no longer pink. Drain off fat.
2. Add oil, onion, and seasonings and stir to mix.
3. Stir in rice and marinara and mix well.
4. Spoon beef mixture into the bell peppers.
5. Place the baking pan in position 2 of the oven. Lightly spray fryer basket with cooking spray.
6. Place peppers in basket and place on baking pan. Set oven to air fry on 355°F for 10 minutes.
7. Remove basket and sprinkle cheese over tops of peppers. Return to oven and cook another 5 minutes, or until peppers are tended and cheese is melted. Serve immediately.
- **Nutrition Info:** Calories 398, Total Fat 16g, Saturated Fat 5g, Total Carbs 35g, Net Carbs 31g, Protein 26g, Sugar 4g, Fiber 4g, Sodium 114mg, Potassium 674mg, Phosphorus 272mg

258.Air Fryer Burgers

Servings: 4
Cooking Time: 10 Minutes
Ingredients:
- 1 pound lean ground beef
- 1 tsp. dried parsley
- ½ tsp. dried oregano
- ½ tsp. pepper
- ½ tsp. salt
- ½ tsp. onion powder
- ½ tsp. garlic powder
- Few drops of liquid smoke
- 1 tsp. Worcestershire sauce

Directions:
1. Preparing the Ingredients. Ensure your air fryer oven is preheated to 350 degrees.
2. Mix all seasonings together till combined.
3. Place beef in a bowl and add seasonings. Mix well, but do not overmix.
4. Make 4 patties from the mixture and using your thumb, making an indent in the center of each patty.
5. Add patties to air fryer rack/basket.
6. Air Frying. Set temperature to 350°F, and set time to 10 minutes, and cook 10 minutes. No need to turn.
- **Nutrition Info:** CALORIES: 148; FAT: 5G; PROTEIN:24G; SUGAR:1G

259.Chicken Wrapped In Bacon

Servings: 2
Cooking Time: 20 Minutes
Ingredients:
- 2 chicken breasts
- 8 oz onion and chive cream cheese
- 1 tbsp butter
- 6 turkey bacon
- Salt to taste
- 1 tbsp fresh parsley, chopped
- Juice from ½ lemon

Directions:
1. Preheat on Air Fry function to 390 F. Stretch out the bacon slightly and lay them in 2 sets; 3 bacon strips together on each side. Place the chicken breast on each bacon set and use a knife to smear cream cheese on both. Share the butter on top and sprinkle with salt. Wrap the bacon around the chicken and secure the ends into the wrap.
2. Place the wrapped chicken in the AirFryer basket and fit in the baking tray; cook for 14 minutes. Turn the chicken halfway through. Remove the chicken to a serving platter and top with parsley and lemon juice. Serve with steamed greens.

260.Balsamic Chicken Breast Roast

Servings:2
Cooking Time: 40 Minutes
Ingredients:
- ¼ cup balsamic vinegar
- 2 teaspoons dried oregano
- 2 garlic cloves, minced
- 1 tablespoon olive oil
- ⅛ teaspoon salt
- ½ teaspoon freshly ground black pepper
- 2 (4-ounce / 113-g) boneless, skinless, chicken-breast halves
- Cooking spray

Directions:
1. In a small bowl, add the vinegar, oregano, garlic, olive oil, salt, and pepper. Mix to combine.
2. Put the chicken in a resealable plastic bag. Pour the vinegar mixture in the bag with the chicken, seal the bag, and shake to coat the chicken. Refrigerate for 30 minutes to marinate.
3. Spritz the baking pan with cooking spray. Put the chicken in the prepared baking pan and pour the marinade over the chicken.
4. Slide the baking pan into Rack Position 1, select Convection Bake, set temperature to 400ºF (205ºC) and set time to 40 minutes.
5. After 20 minutes, remove the pan from the oven. Flip the chicken. Return the pan to the oven and continue cooking.

6. When cooking is complete, the internal temperature of the chicken should registers at least 165ºF (74ºC).
7. Let sit for 5 minutes, then serve.

261.Herb Beef Tips

Servings: 6
Cooking Time: 20 Minutes
Ingredients:
- 2 lbs sirloin steak, cut into 1-inch cubes
- 1/4 tsp red chili flakes
- 1/2 tsp pepper
- 1/2 tsp dried thyme
- 1 tsp onion powder
- 1 tsp dried oregano
- 2 tbsp lemon juice
- 2 tbsp water
- 1/4 cup olive oil
- 1 cup parsley, chopped
- 1 tsp garlic, minced
- 1/2 tsp salt

Directions:
1. Fit the oven with the rack in position
2. Add all ingredients into the zip-lock bag, seal bag shake well and place in the refrigerator for 1 hour.
3. Place marinated steak cubes into the parchment-lined baking pan.
4. Set to bake at 400 F for 25 minutes. After 5 minutes place the baking pan in the preheated oven.
5. Serve and enjoy.
- **Nutrition Info:** Calories 361 Fat 18 g Carbohydrates 1.6 g Sugar 0.4 g Protein 46.3 g Cholesterol 135 mg

262.Coconut Chicken Tenders

Servings: 4
Cooking Time: 20 Minutes
Ingredients:
- 1 lb chicken breast, skinless, boneless & cut into strips
- 1 egg, lightly beaten
- 1/4 cup shredded coconut
- 1/2 cup almond meal
- 1/2 tsp garlic powder
- 1/2 tsp cayenne pepper
- 1 tsp paprika
- 1/4 tsp black pepper
- 1/2 tsp sea salt

Directions:
1. Fit the oven with the rack in position
2. In a shallow dish, mix almond meal, shredded coconut, paprika, cayenne pepper, garlic powder, pepper, and salt.
3. In a separate bowl, whisk the egg.
4. Dip each chicken strip in egg then coat with almond meal mixture,

5. Place coat chicken strips in a parchment-lined baking pan.
6. Set to bake at 400 F for 25 minutes. After 5 minutes place the baking pan in the preheated oven.
7. Serve and enjoy.
- **Nutrition Info:** Calories 235 Fat 11.7 g Carbohydrates 4.2 g Sugar 1.1 g Protein 28.3 g Cholesterol 114 mg

263.Meat Lovers' Pizza

Servings: 2
Cooking Time: 12 Minutes
Ingredients:
- 1 pre-prepared 7-inch pizza pie crust, defrosted if necessary.
- 1/3 cup of marinara sauce.
- 2 ounces of grilled steak, sliced into bite-sized pieces
- 2 ounces of salami, sliced fine
- 2 ounces of pepperoni, sliced fine
- ¼ cup of American cheese
- ¼ cup of shredded mozzarella cheese

Directions:
1. Preparing the Ingredients. Preheat the air fryer oven to 350 degrees. Lay the pizza dough flat on a sheet of parchment paper or tin foil, cut large enough to hold the entire pie crust, but small enough that it will leave the edges of theair frying rack/basket uncovered to allow for air circulation. Using a fork, stab the pizza dough several times across the surface – piercing the pie crust will allow air to circulate throughout the crust and ensure even cooking. With a deep soup spoon, ladle the marinara sauce onto the pizza dough, and spread evenly in expanding circles over the surface of the pie-crust. Be sure to leave at least ½ inch of bare dough around the edges, to ensure that extra-crispy crunchy first bite of the crust! Distribute the pieces of steak and the slices of salami and pepperoni evenly over the sauce-covered dough, then sprinkle the cheese in an even layer on top.
2. Air Frying. Set the air fryer oven timer to 12 minutes, and place the pizza with foil or paper on the fryer's basket surface. Again, be sure to leave the edges of the basket uncovered to allow for proper air circulation, and don't let your bare fingers touch the hot surface. After 12 minutes, when the air fryer oven shuts off, the cheese should be perfectly melted and lightly crisped, and the pie crust should be golden brown. Using a spatula – or two, if necessary, remove the pizza from the Oven rack/basket and set on a serving plate. Wait a few minutes until the pie is cool enough to handle, then cut into slices and serve.

264.Chicken Madeira

Servings:x
Cooking Time:x
Ingredients:
- 2 cups Madeira wine
- 2 cups beef broth
- ½ cup shredded Mozzarella cheese
- 4 boneless, skinless chicken breasts
- 1 Tbsp salt
- Salt and freshly ground black pepper, to taste
- 6 cups water
- ½ lb. asparagus, trimmed
- 2 Tbsp extra-virgin olive oil
- 2 Tbsp chopped fresh parsley

Directions:
1. Lay the chicken breasts on a cutting board, and cover each with a piece of plastic wrap. Use a mallet or a small, heavy frying pan to pound them to ¼ inch thick. Discard the plastic wrap and season with salt and pepper on both sides of the chicken.
2. Fill oven with the water, bring to a boil, and add the salt.
3. Add the asparagus and boil, uncovered, until crisp, tender, and bright green, 2 to 3 minutes. Remove immediately and set aside. Pour out the water.
4. In oven over medium heat, heat the olive oil. Cook the chicken for 4 to 5 minutes on each side. Remove and set aside.
5. Add the Madeira wine and beef broth. Bring to a boil, reduce to a simmer, and cook for 10 to 12 minutes.
6. Return the chicken to the pot, turning it to coat in the sauce.
7. Lay the asparagus and cheese on top of the chicken. Then transfer oven to the oven broiler and broil for 3 to 4 minutes. Garnish with the parsley, if using, and serve.

265.Delicious Lamb Patties

Servings: 4
Cooking Time: 15 Minutes
Ingredients:
- 1 lb ground lamb
- 1 tsp ground coriander
- 1 tsp ground cumin
- 1/4 cup fresh parsley, chopped
- 1/4 cup onion, minced
- 1 tbsp garlic, minced
- 1/4 tsp cayenne pepper
- 1/2 tsp ground allspice
- 1 tsp ground cinnamon
- 1/4 tsp pepper
- 1 tsp kosher salt

Directions:
1. Fit the oven with the rack in position

2. Add all ingredients into the mixing bowl and mix until well combined.
3. Make small patties from meat mixture and place onto the parchment-lined baking pan.
4. Set to bake at 450 F for 20 minutes. After 5 minutes place the baking pan in the preheated oven.
5. Serve and enjoy.
- **Nutrition Info:** Calories 223 Fat 8.5 g Carbohydrates 2.6 g Sugar 0.4 g Protein 32.3 g Cholesterol 102 mg

266.Mayo Chicken Breasts With Basil & Cheese

Servings:4
Cooking Time: 20 Minutes
Ingredients:
- 4 chicken breasts, cubed
- 1 tsp garlic powder
- 1 cup mayonnaise
- Salt and black pepper to taste
- ½ cup cream cheese, softened
- Chopped basil for garnish

Directions:
1. In a bowl, mix cream cheese, mayonnaise, garlic powder, and salt. Add in the chicken and toss to coat. Place the chicken in the basket and Press Start. Cook for 15 minutes at 380 F on AirFry function. Serve garnished with roughly chopped fresh basil.

267.Easy Chicken Fingers

Servings: 12 Chicken Fingers
Cooking Time: 10 Minutes
Ingredients:
- ½ cup all-purpose flour
- 2 cups panko bread crumbs
- 2 tablespoons canola oil
- 1 large egg
- 3 boneless and skinless chicken breasts, each cut into 4 strips
- Kosher salt and freshly ground black pepper, to taste
- Cooking spray

Directions:
1. Spritz the air fryer basket with cooking spray.
2. Pour the flour in a large bowl. Combine the panko and canola oil on a shallow dish. Whisk the egg in a separate bowl.
3. Rub the chicken strips with salt and ground black pepper on a clean work surface, then dip the chicken in the bowl of flour. Shake the excess off and dunk the chicken strips in the bowl of whisked egg, then roll the strips over the panko to coat well.
4. Arrange the strips in the basket.
5. Put the air fryer basket on the baking pan and slide into Rack Position 2, select Air Fry,

set temperature to 360ºF (182ºC) and set time to 10 minutes.
6. Flip the strips halfway through.
7. When cooking is complete, the strips should be crunchy and lightly browned.
8. Serve immediately.

268.Duck Breasts With Marmalade Balsamic Glaze

Servings:4
Cooking Time: 13 Minutes
Ingredients:
- 4 (6-ounce / 170-g) skin-on duck breasts
- 1 teaspoon salt
- ¼ cup orange marmalade
- 1 tablespoon white balsamic vinegar
- ¾ teaspoon ground black pepper

Directions:
1. Cut 10 slits into the skin of the duck breasts, then sprinkle with salt on both sides.
2. Place the breasts in the air fryer basket, skin side up.
3. Put the air fryer basket on the baking pan and slide into Rack Position 2, select Air Fry, set temperature to 400ºF (205ºC) and set time to 10 minutes.
4. Meanwhile, combine the remaining ingredients in a small bowl. Stir to mix well.
5. When cooking is complete, brush the duck skin with the marmalade mixture. Flip the breast and air fry for 3 more minutes or until the skin is crispy and the breast is well browned.
6. Serve immediately.

269.Garlic Chicken Wings

Servings: 2
Cooking Time: 25 Minutes
Ingredients:
- 1 lb chicken wings
- 2 tbsp butter, melted
- 1 tbsp garlic, minced

Directions:
1. Fit the oven with the rack in position 2.
2. In a large bowl, mix butter and garlic. Add chicken wings and toss to coat.
3. Add marinated chicken wings to the air fryer basket then place an air fryer basket in the baking pan.
4. Place a baking pan on the oven rack. Set to air fry at 360 F for 25 minutes.
5. Serve and enjoy.
- **Nutrition Info:** Calories 539 Fat 28.4 g Carbohydrates 1.4 g Sugar 0.1 g Protein 66 g Cholesterol 232 mg

270.Pork Neck With Salad

Servings: 2
Cooking Time: 12 Minutes

Ingredients:

- For Pork:
- 1 tablespoon soy sauce
- 1 tablespoon fish sauce
- ½ tablespoon oyster sauce
- ½ pound pork neck
- For Salad:
- 1 ripe tomato, sliced tickly
- 8-10 Thai shallots, sliced
- 1 scallion, chopped
- 1 bunch fresh basil leaves
- 1 bunch fresh cilantro leaves
- For Dressing:
- 3 tablespoons fish sauce
- 2 tablespoons olive oil
- 1 teaspoon apple cider vinegar
- 1 tablespoon palm sugar
- 2 bird eye chili
- 1 tablespoon garlic, minced

Directions:

1. Preparing the Ingredients. For pork in a bowl, mix together all ingredients except pork.
2. Add pork neck and coat with marinade evenly. Refrigerate for about 2-3 hours.
3. Preheat the air fryer oven to 340 degrees F.
4. Air Frying. Place the pork neck onto a grill pan. Cook for about 12 minutes.
5. Meanwhile, in a large salad bowl, mix together all salad ingredients.
6. In a bowl, add all dressing ingredients and beat till well combined.
7. Remove pork neck from Air fryer oven and cut into desired slices.
8. Place pork slices over salad.

271.Beer Corned Beef With Carrots

Servings:4
Cooking Time: 35 Minutes
Ingredients:

- 1 tbsp beef spice
- 1 white onion, chopped
- 2 carrots, chopped
- 12 oz bottle beer
- 1 ½ cups chicken broth
- 4 pounds corned beef

Directions:

1. Cover beef with beer and let sit in the fridge for 30 minutes. Transfer to a pot over medium heat and add in chicken broth, carrots, and onion. Bring to a boil and simmer for 10 minutes. Drain boiled meat and veggies and place them in a baking dish. Sprinkle with beef spice. Select Bake function, adjust the temperature to 400 F, and press Start. Cook for 30 minutes.

272.Bacon-wrapped And Cheese-stuffed Chicken

Servings:4
Cooking Time: 20 Minutes
Ingredients:

- 4 (5-ounce / 142-g) boneless, skinless chicken breasts, pounded to ¼ inch thick
- 1 cup cream cheese
- 2 tablespoons chopped fresh chives
- 8 slices thin-cut bacon
- Sprig of fresh cilantro, for garnish
- Cooking spray

Directions:

1. Spritz the air fryer basket with cooking spray.
2. On a clean work surface, slice the chicken horizontally to make a 1-inch incision on top of each chicken breast with a knife, then cut into the chicken to make a pocket. Leave a ½-inch border along the sides and bottom.
3. Combine the cream cheese and chives in a bowl. Stir to mix well, then gently pour the mixture into the chicken pockets.
4. Wrap each stuffed chicken breast with 2 bacon slices, then secure the ends with toothpicks.
5. Arrange them in the basket.
6. Put the air fryer basket on the baking pan and slide into Rack Position 2, select Air Fry, set temperature to 400ºF (205ºC) and set time to 20 minutes.
7. Flip the bacon-wrapped chicken halfway through the cooking time.
8. When cooking is complete, the bacon should be browned and crispy.
9. Transfer them on a large plate and serve with cilantro on top.

273.Meatballs(3)

Servings: 4
Cooking Time: 20 Minutes
Ingredients:

- 1 lb ground beef
- 1/2 small onion, chopped
- 1 egg, lightly beaten
- 2 garlic cloves, minced
- 1 tbsp basil, chopped
- 1/4 cup parmesan cheese, grated
- 1/2 cup breadcrumbs
- 1 tbsp Italian parsley, chopped
- 1 tbsp rosemary, chopped
- 2 tbsp milk
- Pepper
- Salt

Directions:

1. Fit the oven with the rack in position
2. Add all ingredients into the mixing bowl and mix until well combined.

3. Make small balls from the meat mixture and place them into the baking pan.
4. Set to bake at 375 F for 25 minutes. After 5 minutes place the baking pan in the preheated oven.
5. Serve and enjoy.
- **Nutrition Info:** Calories 311 Fat 10.4 g Carbohydrates 12.3 g Sugar 1.7 g Protein 39.9 g Cholesterol 147 mg

274.Meatballs(13)

Servings: 4
Cooking Time: 20 Minutes
Ingredients:
- 1 lb ground turkey
- 1/4 cup basil, chopped
- 3 tbsp scallions, chopped
- 1 egg, lightly beaten
- 1/2 cup almond flour
- 1/2 tsp red pepper, crushed
- 1 tbsp lemongrass, chopped
- 1 1/2 tbsp fish sauce
- 2 garlic cloves, minced

Directions:
1. Fit the oven with the rack in position 2.
2. Line the air fryer basket with parchment paper.
3. Add all ingredients into a large bowl and mix until well combined.
4. Make small balls from meat mixture and place in the air fryer basket then place the air fryer basket in the baking pan.
5. Place a baking pan on the oven rack. Set to air fry at 380 F for 20 minutes.
6. Serve and enjoy.
- **Nutrition Info:** Calories 269 Fat 15.4 g Carbohydrates 3.4 g Sugar 1.3 g Protein 33.9 g Cholesterol 157 mg

275.Chicken Wings With Buffalo Sauce

Servings:4
Cooking Time: 35 Minutes
Ingredients:
- 2 pounds chicken wing
- ½ cup cayenne pepper sauce
- 2 tbsp coconut oil
- 1 tbsp Worcestershire sauce
- 1 tbsp kosher salt

Directions:
1. In a bowl, combine cayenne pepper sauce, coconut oil, Worcestershire sauce, and salt. Place the chicken in the basket and press Start. Cook for 25 minutes at 380 F on Air Fy function. Increase the temperature to 400 F and cook for 5 more minutes. Transfer into a large-sized bowl and toss in the prepared sauce. Serve with celery sticks and enjoy!

276.Cracker Apple Chicken

Servings: 2
Cooking Time: 45 Minutes
Ingredients:
- 2 chicken breasts, skinless and boneless
- 1 apple, sliced
- 12 Ritz cracker, crushed
- 10 oz can condensed cheddar cheese soup
- Pepper
- Salt

Directions:
1. Fit the oven with the rack in position
2. Season chicken with pepper and salt and place into the baking dish.
3. Arrange sliced apple on top of chicken.
4. Sprinkle crushed crackers on top.
5. Set to bake at 350 F for 50 minutes. After 5 minutes place the baking dish in the preheated oven.
6. Pour cheddar cheese soup on top and serve.
- **Nutrition Info:** Calories 924 Fat 38.2 g Carbohydrates 87 g Sugar 21.4 g Protein 51.8 g Cholesterol 136 mg

277.Baked Fajita Chicken

Servings: 4
Cooking Time: 35 Minutes
Ingredients:
- 4 chicken breasts, sliced
- 2 cups cheddar cheese, shredded
- 2 bell peppers, sliced
- 1 oz fajita seasoning
- 1/3 cup salsa
- 8 oz cream cheese, softened

Directions:
1. Fit the oven with the rack in position
2. Place chicken into the greased 9*13-inch baking dish.
3. Mix together salsa, cream cheese, and fajita seasoning and pour over chicken.
4. Spread sliced bell peppers on top of chicken. Sprinkle shredded cheese on top.
5. Set to bake at 375 F for 40 minutes. After 5 minutes place the baking dish in the preheated oven.
6. Serve and enjoy.
- **Nutrition Info:** Calories 754 Fat 49.5 g Carbohydrates 252 g Sugar 4.1 g Protein 61.5 g Cholesterol 252 mg

278.Dijon Garlic Pork Tenderloin

Servings: 6
Cooking Time: 10 Minutes
Ingredients:
- 1 C. breadcrumbs
- Pinch of cayenne pepper
- 3 crushed garlic cloves
- 2 tbsp. ground ginger
- 2 tbsp. Dijon mustard

- 2 tbsp. raw honey
- 4 tbsp. water
- 2 tsp. salt
- 1 pound pork tenderloin, sliced into 1-inch rounds

Directions:
1. Preparing the Ingredients. With pepper and salt, season all sides of tenderloin.
2. Combine cayenne pepper, garlic, ginger, mustard, honey, and water until smooth.
3. Dip pork rounds into the honey mixture and then into breadcrumbs, ensuring they all get coated well.
4. Place coated pork rounds into your air fryer oven.
5. Air Frying. Set temperature to 400°F, and set time to 10 minutes. Cook 10 minutes at 400 degrees. Flip and then cook an additional 5 minutes until golden in color.
- **Nutrition Info:** CALORIES: 423; FAT: 18G; PROTEIN:31G; SUGAR:3G

279.Mutton Fried Baked Pastry

Servings:x
Cooking Time:x
Ingredients:
- A small amount of ginger either grated or finely chopped
- 1 or 2 green chilies that are finely chopped or mashed
- ½ tsp cumin
- 1 tsp coarsely crushed whole coriander
- 1 dry red chili broken into pieces
- A small amount of salt
- 2 tbsp. unsalted butter
- 1 ½ cup all-purpose flour
- A pinch of salt to taste
- Add as much water as required to make the dough stiff and firm
- For filling:
- 2 cups minced mutton
- ¼ cup boiled peas
- ½ tsp dried mango powder
- ½ tsp red chili power
- 1-2 tbsp. coriander

Directions:
1. You will first need to make the outer covering. In a large bowl, add the flour, butter and enough water to knead it into dough that is stiff. Transfer this to a container and leave it to rest for five minutes. Place a pan on medium flame and add the oil. Roast the mustard seeds and once roasted, add the coriander seeds and the chopped dry red chilies. Add all the dry ingredients for the filling and mix the ingredients well. Add a little water and continue to stir the ingredients. Make small balls out of the dough and roll them out.

2. Cut the rolled-out dough into halves and apply a little water on the edges to help you fold the halves into a cone. Add the filling to the cone and close up the samosa. Pre-heat the oven for around 5 to 6 minutes at 300 Fahrenheit. Place all the samosas in the fry basket and close the basket properly. Keep the oven at 200 degrees for another 20 to 25 minutes. Around the halfway point, open the basket and turn the samosas over for uniform cooking. After this, fry at 250 degrees for around 10 minutes in order to give them the desired golden-brown color. Serve hot. Recommended sides are tamarind or mint sauce.

280.Greek Chicken Breast

Servings: 4
Cooking Time: 25 Minutes
Ingredients:
- 4 chicken breasts, skinless & boneless
- 1 tbsp olive oil
- For rub:
- 1 tsp oregano
- 1 tsp thyme
- 1 tsp parsley
- 1 tsp onion powder
- 1 tsp basil
- Pepper
- Salt

Directions:
1. Fit the oven with the rack in position 2.
2. Brush chicken with olive oil.
3. In a small bowl, mix together all rub ingredients and rub all over the chicken breasts.
4. Place chicken into the air fryer basket then places the air fryer basket in the baking pan.
5. Place a baking pan on the oven rack. Set to air fry at 390 F for 25 minutes.
6. Serve and enjoy.
- **Nutrition Info:** Calories 312 Fat 14.4 g Carbohydrates 0.9 g Sugar 0.2 g Protein 42.4 g Cholesterol 130 mg

281.Comforting Red Wine Steak

Servings:x
Cooking Time:x
Ingredients:
- 2 (8-oz) sirloin steaks, trimmed of fat
- Salt and freshly ground black pepper, to taste
- 4 Tbsp extra-virgin olive oil, divided
- 1 lb. fingerling potatoes, rinsed, halved
- 3 Tbsp shallots, minced
- 2 tsp chopped fresh thyme
- ¾ cup red wine

Directions:

1. Pat the steaks dry with a paper towel. Season generously with salt and pepper. Let them rest at room temperature for 15 to 20 minutes before cooking.
2. In oven over medium heat, heat 1 Tbsp of olive oil.
3. Add the potatoes, season with salt and pepper, and toss. Cook covered over low heat for 20 to 30 minutes. Set aside.
4. Heat oven over high heat. Add the remaining 3 Tbsp of oil, then lower the heat to medium-high.
5. Add the steaks and cook for 4 minutes on each side for medium-rare, or longer as desired. Remove from the pot and set aside.
6. Add the shallots and thyme to the pot.
7. Add the wine and cook until the liquid is almost evaporated, 1 to 2 minutes. Season with salt and pepper, and stir with a whisk.
8. Spoon the sauce over the steaks, and serve with the potatoes.

282.Air Fryer Herb Pork Chops

Servings: 4
Cooking Time: 15 Minutes
Ingredients:
- 4 pork chops
- 2 tsp oregano
- 2 tsp thyme
- 2 tsp sage
- 1 tsp garlic powder
- 1 tsp paprika
- 1 tsp rosemary
- Pepper
- Salt

Directions:
1. Fit the oven with the rack in position 2.
2. Line the air fryer basket with parchment paper.
3. Mix garlic powder, paprika, rosemary, oregano, thyme, sage, pepper, and salt and rub over pork chops.
4. Place pork chops in the air fryer basket then place an air fryer basket in the baking pan.
5. Place a baking pan on the oven rack. Set to air fry at 360 F for 15 minutes.
6. Serve and enjoy.
- **Nutrition Info:** Calories 266 Fat 20.2 g Carbohydrates 2 g Sugar 0.3 g Protein 18.4 g Cholesterol 69 mg

283.Basil Mozzarella Chicken

Servings: 4
Cooking Time: 25 Minutes
Ingredients:
- 4 chicken breasts, cubed
- 4 basil leaves
- ¼ cup balsamic vinegar
- 4 slices tomato
- 1 tbsp butter
- 4 slices mozzarella cheese

Directions:
1. Heat butter and balsamic vinegar in a pan over medium heat. Pour over the chicken. Place the chicken in a baking pan and cook for 20 minutes at 400 F on Bake function. Top with cheese, and Bake for 1 minute until the cheese melts. Cover with basil and tomato slices and serve.

284.Beef Rolls With Pesto & Spinach

Servings: 4
Cooking Time: 30 Minutes
Ingredients:
- 2 pounds beef steaks, sliced
- Salt and black pepper to taste
- 3 tbsp pesto
- 6 slices mozzarella cheese
- ¾ cup spinach, chopped
- 3 oz bell pepper, deseeded and sliced

Directions:
1. Top the meat with pesto, mozzarella cheese, spinach, and bell pepper. Roll up the slices and secure using a toothpick. Season with salt and pepper. Place the slices in the basket and fit in the baking tray; cook for 15 minutes on Air Fry function at 400 F, turning once. Serve immediately!

285.Spiced Pork Roast

Servings: 8
Cooking Time: 50 Minutes
Ingredients:
- Nonstick cooking spray
- 3 1/3 tbsp. brown sugar
- 2/3 tbsp. sugar
- 1 ½ tsp pepper
- 1 tsp salt
- 1 tsp ginger
- ¾ tsp garlic powder
- ¾ tsp onion salt
- ½ tbsp. dry mustard
- ¼ tsp cayenne pepper
- ¼ tsp crushed red pepper flakes
- ¼ tsp cumin
- ¼ tsp paprika
- ¾ tsp thyme
- 2 ½ lb. pork loin roast, boneless

Directions:
1. Place baking pan in position 1 of the oven. Spray the fryer basket with cooking spray.
2. In a small bowl, combine sugars and spices, mix well.
3. Rub spice mixture into all sides of the pork roast. Place roast in the basket.
4. Set oven to convection bake on 300°F for 60 minutes. After 5 minutes, place the basket on the pan and cook 45-50 minutes.

5. Remove from oven and let rest 10 minutes before slicing and serving.
- **Nutrition Info:** Calories 224, Total Fat 6g, Saturated Fat 2g, Total Carbs 8g, Net Carbs 8g, Protein 32g, Sugar 8g, Fiber 0g, Sodium 362mg, Potassium 549mg, Phosphorus 321mg

FISH & SEAFOOD RECIPES

286.Fish Cakes With Mango Relish

Servings: 4
Cooking Time: 10 Minutes
Ingredients:
- 1 lb White Fish Fillets
- 3 Tbsps Ground Coconut
- 1 Ripened Mango
- ½ Tsps Chili Paste
- Tbsps Fresh Parsley
- 1 Green Onion
- 1 Lime
- 1 Tsp Salt
- 1 Egg

Directions:
1. Preparing the Ingredients. To make the relish, peel and dice the mango into cubes. Combine with a half teaspoon of chili paste, a tablespoon of parsley, and the zest and juice of half a lime.
2. In a food processor, pulse the fish until it forms a smooth texture. Place into a bowl and add the salt, egg, chopped green onion, parsley, two tablespoons of the coconut, and the remainder of the chili paste and lime zest and juice. Combine well
3. Portion the mixture into 10 equal balls and flatten them into small patties. Pour the reserved tablespoon of coconut onto a dish and roll the patties over to coat.
4. Preheat the Air fryer oven to 390 degrees
5. Air Frying. Place the fish cakes into the air fryer oven and cook for 8 minutes. They should be crisp and lightly browned when ready
6. Serve hot with mango relish

287.Tomato Garlic Shrimp

Servings: 4
Cooking Time: 25 Minutes
Ingredients:
- 1 lb shrimp, peeled
- 1 tbsp garlic, sliced
- 2 cups cherry tomatoes
- 1 tbsp olive oil
- Pepper
- Salt

Directions:
1. Fit the oven with the rack in position
2. Add shrimp, oil, garlic, tomatoes, pepper, and salt into the large bowl and toss well.
3. Transfer shrimp mixture into the baking dish.
4. Set to bake at 400 F for 30 minutes. After 5 minutes place the baking dish in the preheated oven.
5. Serve and enjoy.

- **Nutrition Info:** Calories 184 Fat 5.6 g Carbohydrates 5.9 g Sugar 2.4 g Protein 26.8 gCholesterol 239 mg

288.Baked Tilapia

Servings: 4
Cooking Time: 10 Minutes
Ingredients:
- 1 1/4 lbs tilapia fillets
- 2 tsp onion powder
- 2 tbsp olive oil
- 1/2 tsp garlic powder
- 1/2 tsp dried thyme
- 1/2 tsp oregano
- 1/2 tsp chili powder
- 2 tbsp sweet paprika
- 1 tsp pepper
- 1/2 tsp salt

Directions:
1. Fit the oven with the rack in position
2. Brush fish fillets with oil and place in baking dish.
3. Mix together spices and sprinkle over the fish fillets.
4. Set to bake at 425 F for 15 minutes. After 5 minutes place the baking dish in the preheated oven.
5. Serve and enjoy.
- **Nutrition Info:** Calories 195 Fat 8.9 g Carbohydrates 3.9 g Sugar 0.9 g Protein 27.2 g Cholesterol 69 mg

289.Harissa Shrimp

Servings:4
Cooking Time: 15 Minutes
Ingredients:
- 1 ¼ lb tiger shrimp
- ¼ tsp harissa powder
- ½ tsp old bay seasoning
- Salt to taste
- 1 tbsp olive oil

Directions:
1. Preheat your oven to 390 F on AirFry function. In a bowl, mix the ingredients. Place the mixture in the cooking basket and cook for 5 minutes. Serve with a drizzle of lemon juice.

290.Cajun Red Snapper

Servings: 2
Cooking Time: 12 Minutes
Ingredients:
- 8 oz red snapper fillets
- 2 tbsp parmesan cheese, grated
- 1/4 cup breadcrumbs
- 1/2 tsp Cajun seasoning
- 1/4 tsp Worcestershire sauce

- 1 garlic clove, minced
- 1/4 cup butter

Directions:
1. Fit the oven with the rack in position
2. Melt butter in a pan over low heat. Add Cajun seasoning, garlic, and Worcestershire sauce into the melted butter and stir well.
3. Brush fish fillets with melted butter and place into the baking dish.
4. Mix together parmesan cheese and breadcrumbs and sprinkle over fish fillets.
5. Set to bake at 400 F for 17 minutes. After 5 minutes place the baking dish in the preheated oven.
6. Serve and enjoy.
- **Nutrition Info:** Calories 424 Fat 27 g Carbohydrates 10.6 g Sugar 1 g Protein 33.9 g Cholesterol 119 mg

291.Salmon Beans & Mushrooms

Servings: 6
Cooking Time: 25 Minutes
Ingredients:
- 4 salmon fillets
- 2 tbsp fresh parsley, minced
- 1/4 cup fresh lemon juice
- 1 tsp garlic, minced
- 1 tbsp olive oil
- 1/2 lb mushrooms, sliced
- 1/2 lb green beans, trimmed
- 1/2 cup parmesan cheese, grated
- Pepper
- Salt

Directions:
1. Fit the oven with the rack in position
2. Heat oil in a small saucepan over medium-high heat.
3. Add garlic and sauté for 30 seconds.
4. Remove from heat and stir in lemon juice, parsley, pepper, and salt.
5. Arrange fish fillets, mushrooms, and green beans in baking pan and drizzle with oil mixture.
6. Sprinkle with grated parmesan cheese.
7. Set to bake at 400 F for 30 minutes. After 5 minutes place the baking pan in the preheated oven.
8. Serve and enjoy.
- **Nutrition Info:** Calories 225 Fat 11.5 g Carbohydrates 4.7 g Sugar 1.4 g Protein 27.5 g Cholesterol 58 mg

292.Baked Lemon Swordfish

Servings: 2
Cooking Time: 10 Minutes
Ingredients:
- 12 oz swordfish fillets
- 1/8 tsp crushed red pepper
- 1 garlic clove, minced

- 2 tsp fresh parsley, chopped
- 3 tbsp olive oil
- 1/2 tsp lemon zest, grated
- 1/2 tsp ginger, grated

Directions:
1. Fit the oven with the rack in position
2. In a small bowl, mix 2 tbsp oil, lemon zest, red pepper, ginger, garlic, and parsley.
3. Season fish fillets with salt.
4. Heat remaining oil in a pan over medium-high heat.
5. Place fish fillets in the pan and cook until browned, about 2-3 minutes.
6. Transfer fish fillets in a baking dish.
7. Set to bake at 400 F for 15 minutes. After 5 minutes place the baking dish in the preheated oven.
8. Pour oil mixture over fish fillets and serve.
- **Nutrition Info:** Calories 449 Fat 29.8 g Carbohydrates 1.1 g Sugar 0.1 g Protein 43.4 g Cholesterol 85 mg

293.Seafood Mac N Cheese

Servings: 8
Cooking Time: 30 Minutes
Ingredients:
- Nonstick cooking spray
- 16 oz. macaroni
- 7 tbsp. butter, divided
- ¾ lb. medium shrimp, peel, devein, & cut in ½-inch pieces
- ½ cup Italian panko bread crumbs
- 1 cup onion, chopped fine
- 1 ½ tsp garlic, diced fine
- 1/3 cup flour
- 3 cups milk
- 1/8 tsp nutmeg
- ½ tsp Old Bay seasoning
- 1 tsp salt
- ¾ tsp pepper
- 1 1/3 cup Parmesan cheese, grated
- 1 1/3 cup Swiss cheese, grated
- 1 1/3 cup sharp cheddar cheese, grated
- ½ lb. lump crab meat, cooked

Directions:
1. Place wire rack in position 1 of the oven. Spray a 7x11-inch baking dish with cooking spray.
2. Cook macaroni according to package directions, shortening cooking time by 2 minutes. Drain and rinse with cold water.
3. Melt 1 tablespoon butter in a large skillet over med-high heat. Add shrimp and cook, stirring, until they turn pink. Remove from heat.
4. Melt remaining butter in a large saucepan over medium heat. Once melted, transfer 2 tablespoons to a small bowl and mix in bread crumbs.

5. Add onions and garlic to saucepan and cook, stirring, until they soften.
6. Whisk in flour and cook 1 minute, until smooth.
7. Whisk in milk until there are no lumps. Bring to a boil, reduce heat and simmer until thickened, whisking constantly.
8. Whisk in seasonings. Stir in cheese until melted and smooth. Fold in macaroni and seafood. Transfer to prepared dish. Sprinkle bread crumb mixture evenly over top.
9. Set oven to bake on 400°F for 25 minutes. After 5 minutes, place dish on the rack and bake 20 minutes, until topping is golden brown and sauce is bubbly. Let cool 5 minutes before serving.
- **Nutrition Info:** Calories 672, Total Fat 26g, Saturated Fat 15g, Total Carbs 68g, Net Carbs 61g, Protein 39g, Sugar 7g, Fiber 7g, Sodium 996mg, Potassium 921mg, Phosphorus 714mg

294.Seafood Pizza

Servings:x
Cooking Time:x
Ingredients:
- One pizza base
- Grated pizza cheese (mozzarella cheese preferably) for topping
- Some pizza topping sauce
- Use cooking oil for brushing and topping purposes
- ingredients for topping:
- 2 onions chopped
- 2 cups mixed seafood
- 2 capsicums chopped
- 2 tomatoes that have been deseeded and chopped
- 1 tbsp. (optional) mushrooms/corns
- 2 tsp. pizza seasoning
- Some cottage cheese that has been cut into small cubes (optional)

Directions:
1. Put the pizza base in a pre-heated oven for around 5 minutes. (Pre heated to 340 Fahrenheit). Take out the base. Pour some pizza sauce on top of the base at the center. Using a spoon spread the sauce over the base making sure that you leave some gap around the circumference. Grate some mozzarella cheese and sprinkle it over the sauce layer. Take all the vegetables and the seafood and mix them in a bowl. Add some oil and seasoning.
2. Also add some salt and pepper according to taste. Mix them properly. Put this topping over the layer of cheese on the pizza. Now sprinkle some more grated cheese and pizza seasoning on top of this layer. Pre

heat the oven at 250 Fahrenheit for around 5 minutes.
3. Open the fry basket and place the pizza inside. Close the basket and keep the fryer at 170 degrees for another 10 minutes. If you feel that it is undercooked you may put it at the same temperature for another 2 minutes or so.

295.Prawn Fried Baked Pastry

Servings:x
Cooking Time:x
Ingredients:
- 2 tbsp. unsalted butter
- 1 ½ cup all-purpose flour
- A pinch of salt to taste
- Add as much water as required to make the dough stiff and firm
- 1 lb. prawn
- ¼ cup boiled peas
- 1 tsp. powdered ginger
- 1 or 2 green chilies that are finely chopped or mashed
- ½ tsp. cumin
- 1 tsp. coarsely crushed coriander
- 1 dry red chili broken into pieces
- A small amount of salt (to taste)
- ½ tsp. dried mango powder
- ½ tsp. red chili power.
- 1-2 tbsp. coriander.

Directions:
1. You will first need to make the outer covering. In a large bowl, add the flour, butter and enough water to knead it into dough that is stiff. Transfer this to a container and leave it to rest for five minutes. Place a pan on medium flame and add the oil. Roast the mustard seeds and once roasted, add the coriander seeds and the chopped dry red chilies. Add all the dry ingredients for the filling and mix the ingredients well.
2. Add a little water and continue to stir the ingredients. Make small balls out of the dough and roll them out. Cut the rolled-out dough into halves and apply a little water on the edges to help you fold the halves into a cone. Add the filling to the cone and close up the samosa. Pre-heat the oven for around 5 to 6 minutes at 300 Fahrenheit. Place all the samosas in the fry basket and close the basket properly.
3. Keep the oven at 200 degrees for another 20 to 25 minutes. Around the halfway point, open the basket and turn the samosas over for uniform cooking. After this, fry at 250 degrees for around 10 minutes in order to give them the desired golden-brown color.

Serve hot. Recommended sides are tamarind or mint sauce.

296.Cajun And Lemon Pepper Cod

Servings: 2 Cod Fillets
Cooking Time: 12 Minutes
Ingredients:
- 1 tablespoon Cajun seasoning
- 1 teaspoon salt
- ½ teaspoon lemon pepper
- ½ teaspoon freshly ground black pepper
- 2 (8-ounce / 227-g) cod fillets, cut to fit into the air fryer basket
- Cooking spray
- 2 tablespoons unsalted butter, melted
- 1 lemon, cut into 4 wedges

Directions:
1. Spritz the baking pan with cooking spray.
2. Thoroughly combine the Cajun seasoning, salt, lemon pepper, and black pepper in a small bowl. Rub this mixture all over the cod fillets until completely coated.
3. Put the fillets in the prepared pan and brush the melted butter over both sides of each fillet.
4. Slide the baking pan into Rack Position 1, select Convection Bake, set temperature to 360ºF (182ºC), and set time to 12 minutes.
5. Flip the fillets halfway through the cooking time.
6. When cooking is complete, the fish should flake apart with a fork. Remove the fillets from the oven and serve with fresh lemon wedges.

297.Mediterranean Sole

Servings: 6
Cooking Time: 20 Minutes
Ingredients:
- Nonstick cooking spray
- 2 tbsp. olive oil
- 8 scallions, sliced thin
- 2 cloves garlic, diced fine
- 4 tomatoes, chopped
- ½ cup dry white wine
- 2 tbsp. fresh parsley, chopped fine
- 1 tsp oregano
- 1 tsp pepper
- 2 lbs. sole, cut in 6 pieces
- 4 oz. feta cheese, crumbled

Directions:
1. Place the rack in position 1 of the oven. Spray an 8x11-inch baking dish with cooking spray.
2. Heat the oil in a medium skillet over medium heat. Add scallions and garlic and cook until tender, stirring frequently.
3. Add the tomatoes, wine, parsley, oregano, and pepper. Stir to mix. Simmer for 5

minutes, or until sauce thickens. Remove from heat.
4. Pour half the sauce on the bottom of the prepared dish. Lay fish on top then pour remaining sauce over the top. Sprinkle with feta.
5. Set the oven to bake on 400°F for 25 minutes. After 5 minutes, place the baking dish on the rack and cook 15-18 minutes or until fish flakes easily with a fork. Serve immediately.
- **Nutrition Info:** Calories 220, Total Fat 12g, Saturated Fat 4g, Total Carbs 6g, Net Carbs 4g, Protein 22g, Sugar 4g, Fiber 2g, Sodium 631mg, Potassium 540mg, Phosphorus 478mg

298.Carp Flat Cakes

Servings:x
Cooking Time:x
Ingredients:
- 2 tbsp. garam masala
- 1 lb. fileted carp
- 3 tsp ginger finely chopped
- 1-2 tbsp. fresh coriander leaves
- 2 or 3 green chilies finely chopped
- 1 ½ tbsp. lemon juice
- Salt and pepper to taste

Directions:
1. Mix the ingredients in a clean bowl and add water to it. Make sure that the paste is not too watery but is enough to apply on the sides of the carp filets.
2. Pre heat the oven at 160 degrees Fahrenheit for 5 minutes. Place the French Cuisine Galettes in the fry basket and let them cook for another 25 minutes at the same temperature. Keep rolling them over to get a uniform cook. Serve either with mint sauce or ketchup.

299.Carp Fritters

Servings:x
Cooking Time:x
Ingredients:
- 10 carp filets
- 3 onions chopped
- 5 green chilies-roughly chopped
- 1 ½ tbsp. ginger paste
- 1 ½ tsp. garlic paste
- 1 ½ tsp. salt
- 3 tsp. lemon juice
- 2 tsp. garam masala
- 3 eggs
- 2 ½ tbsp. white sesame seeds

Directions:
1. Grind the ingredients except for the egg and form a smooth paste. Coat the filets in the

paste. Now, beat the eggs and add a little salt to it.

2. Dip the coated filets in the egg mixture and then transfer to the sesame seeds and coat the florets well. Place the vegetables on a stick.

3. Pre heat the oven at 160 degrees Fahrenheit for around 5 minutes. Place the sticks in the basket and let them cook for another 25 minutes at the same temperature. Turn the sticks over in between the cooking process to get a uniform cook.

300.Fried Calamari

Servings: 6-8
Cooking Time: 7 Minutes
Ingredients:
- ½ tsp. salt
- ½ tsp. Old Bay seasoning
- 1/3 C. plain cornmeal
- ½ C. semolina flour
- ½ C. almond flour
- 5-6 C. olive oil
- 1 ½ pounds baby squid

Directions:
1. Preparing the Ingredients. Rinse squid in cold water and slice tentacles, keeping just ¼-inch of the hood in one piece.
2. Combine 1-2 pinches of pepper, salt, Old Bay seasoning, cornmeal, and both flours together. Dredge squid pieces into flour mixture and place into the air fryer oven.
3. Air Frying. Spray liberally with olive oil. Cook 15 minutes at 345 degrees till coating turns a golden brown.
- **Nutrition Info:** CALORIES: 211; CARBS:55; FAT: 6G; PROTEIN:21G; SUGAR:1G

301.Cajun Salmon With Lemon

Servings:1
Cooking Time: 10 Minutes
Ingredients:
- 1 salmon fillet
- ¼ tsp brown sugar
- Juice of ½ lemon
- 1 tbsp cajun seasoning
- 2 lemon wedges
- 1 tbsp fresh parsley, chopped

Directions:
1. Preheat on Bake function to 350 F. Combine sugar and lemon and coat in the salmon. Sprinkle with the Cajun seasoning as well. Place a parchment paper on a baking tray and press Start. Cook for 14-16 minutes. Serve with lemon wedges and chopped parsley.

302.Soy And Ginger Shrimp

Servings: 4
Cooking Time: 10 Minutes
Ingredients:
- 2 tablespoons olive oil
- 2 tablespoons scallions, finely chopped
- 2 cloves garlic, chopped
- 1 teaspoon fresh ginger, grated
- 1 tablespoon dry white wine
- 1 tablespoon balsamic vinegar
- 1/4 cup soy sauce
- 1 tablespoon sugar
- 1 pound shrimp
- Salt and ground black pepper, to taste

Directions:
1. Preparing the Ingredients. To make the marinade, warm the oil in a saucepan; cook all ingredients, except the shrimp, salt, and black pepper. Now, let it cool.
2. Marinate the shrimp, covered, at least an hour, in the refrigerator.
3. Air Frying. After that, bake the shrimp at 350 degrees F for 8 to 10 minutes (depending on the size), turning once or twice. Season prepared shrimp with salt and black pepper and serve right away.

303.Easy Blackened Shrimp

Servings: 6
Cooking Time: 10 Minutes
Ingredients:
- 1 lb shrimp, deveined
- 1 tbsp olive oil
- 1/4 tsp pepper
- 2 tsp blackened seasoning
- 1/4 tsp salt

Directions:
1. Fit the oven with the rack in position
2. Toss shrimp with oil, pepper, blackened seasoning, and salt.
3. Transfer shrimp into the baking pan.
4. Set to bake at 400 F for 15 minutes. After 5 minutes place the baking pan in the preheated oven.
5. Serve and enjoy.
- **Nutrition Info:** Calories 167 Fat 4.3 g Carbohydrates 10.5 g Sugar 0 g Protein 20.6 g Cholesterol 159 mg

304.Herb Fish Fillets

Servings: 2
Cooking Time: 5 Minutes
Ingredients:
- 2 salmon fillets
- 1/4 tsp smoked paprika
- 1 tsp herb de Provence
- 1 tbsp butter, melted
- 2 tbsp olive oil

- Pepper
- Salt

Directions:
1. Fit the oven with the rack in position 2.
2. Brush salmon fillets with oil and sprinkle with paprika, herb de Provence, pepper, and salt.
3. Place salmon fillets in the air fryer basket then place an air fryer basket in the baking pan.
4. Place a baking pan on the oven rack. Set to air fry at 390 F for 5 minutes.
5. Drizzle melted butter over salmon and serve.
- **Nutrition Info:** Calories 413 Fat 31.1 g Carbohydrates 0.2 g Sugar 0 g Protein 35.4 g Cholesterol 94 mg

305.Old Bay Shrimp

Servings:4
Cooking Time: 10 Minutes
Ingredients:
- 1 lb jumbo shrimp
- Salt to taste
- ¼ tsp old bay seasoning
- ⅓ tsp smoked paprika
- ¼ tsp chili powder
- 1 tbsp olive oil

Directions:
1. Preheat on AirFry function to 390 F. In a bowl, add the shrimp, paprika, oil, salt, old bay seasoning, and chili powder; mix well. Place the shrimp in the oven and cook for 5 minutes.

306.Herbed Salmon With Asparagus

Servings: 2
Cooking Time: 12 Minutes
Ingredients:
- 2 teaspoons olive oil, plus additional for drizzling
- 2 (5-ounce / 142-g) salmon fillets, with skin
- Salt and freshly ground black pepper, to taste
- 1 bunch asparagus, trimmed
- 1 teaspoon dried tarragon
- 1 teaspoon dried chives
- Fresh lemon wedges, for serving

Directions:
1. Rub the olive oil all over the salmon fillets. Sprinkle with salt and pepper to taste.
2. Put the asparagus on the foil-lined baking pan and place the salmon fillets on top, skin-side down.
3. Slide the baking pan into Rack Position 1, select Convection Bake, set temperature to 350ºF (180ºC), and set time to 12 minutes.
4. When cooked, the fillets should register 145ºF (63ºC) on an instant-read

thermometer. Remove from the oven and cut the salmon fillets in half crosswise, then use a metal spatula to lift flesh from skin and transfer to a serving plate. Discard the skin and drizzle the salmon fillets with additional olive oil. Scatter with the herbs.
5. Serve the salmon fillets with asparagus spears and lemon wedges on the side.

307.Spiced Red Snapper

Servings:4
Cooking Time: 10 Minutes
Ingredients:
- 1 teaspoon olive oil
- 1½ teaspoons black pepper
- ¼ teaspoon garlic powder
- ¼ teaspoon thyme
- ⅛ teaspoon cayenne pepper
- 4 (4-ounce / 113-g) red snapper fillets, skin on
- 4 thin slices lemon
- Nonstick cooking spray

Directions:
1. Spritz the baking pan with nonstick cooking spray.
2. In a small bowl, stir together the olive oil, black pepper, garlic powder, thyme, and cayenne pepper. Rub the mixture all over the fillets until completely coated.
3. Lay the fillets, skin-side down, in the baking pan and top each fillet with a slice of lemon.
4. Slide the baking pan into Rack Position 1, select Convection Bake, set temperature to 390ºF (199ºC), and set time to 10 minutes.
5. Flip the fillets halfway through the cooking time.
6. When cooking is complete, the fish should be cooked through. Let the fish cool for 5 minutes and serve.

308.Spicy Orange Shrimp

Servings:4
Cooking Time: 12 Minutes
Ingredients:
- $^1/_3$ cup orange juice
- 3 teaspoons minced garlic
- 1 teaspoon Old Bay seasoning
- ¼ to ½ teaspoon cayenne pepper
- 1 pound (454 g) medium shrimp, thawed, deveined, peeled, with tails off, and patted dry
- Cooking spray

Directions:
1. Stir together the orange juice, garlic, Old Bay seasoning, and cayenne pepper in a medium bowl. Add the shrimp to the bowl and toss to coat well.
2. Cover the bowl with plastic wrap and marinate in the refrigerator for 30 minutes.

3. Spritz the air fryer basket with cooking spray. Place the shrimp in the pan and spray with cooking spray.
4. Put the air fryer basket on the baking pan and slide into Rack Position 2, select Air Fry, set temperature to 400ºF (205ºC), and set time to 12 minutes.
5. Flip the shrimp halfway through the cooking time.
6. When cooked, the shrimp should be opaque and crisp. Remove from the oven and serve hot.

309.Garlicky Cod Fillets

Servings:4
Cooking Time: 12 Minutes
Ingredients:
- 1 teaspoon olive oil
- 4 cod fillets
- ¼ teaspoon fine sea salt
- ¼ teaspoon ground black pepper, or more to taste
- 1 teaspoon cayenne pepper
- ½ cup fresh Italian parsley, coarsely chopped
- ½ cup nondairy milk
- 1 Italian pepper, chopped
- 4 garlic cloves, minced
- 1 teaspoon dried basil
- ½ teaspoon dried oregano

Directions:
1. Lightly coat the sides and bottom of the baking pan with the olive oil. Set aside.
2. In a large bowl, sprinkle the fillets with salt, black pepper, and cayenne pepper.
3. In a food processor, pulse the remaining ingredients until smoothly puréed.
4. Add the purée to the bowl of fillets and toss to coat, then transfer to the prepared baking pan.
5. Slide the baking pan into Rack Position 1, select Convection Bake, set temperature to 380ºF (193ºC), and set time to 12 minutes.
6. When cooking is complete, the fish should flake when pressed lightly with a fork. Remove from the oven and serve warm.

310.Sesame Seeds Coated Fish

Servings:5
Cooking Time: 8 Minutes
Ingredients:
- 3 tablespoons plain flour
- 2 eggs
- ½ cup sesame seeds, toasted
- ½ cup breadcrumbs
- 1/8 teaspoon dried rosemary, crushed
- Pinch of salt
- Pinch of black pepper
- 3 tablespoons olive oil

- 5 frozen fish fillets (white fish of your choice)

Directions:
1. Preparing the Ingredients. In a shallow dish, place flour. In a second shallow dish, beat the eggs. In a third shallow dish, add remaining ingredients except fish fillets and mix till a crumbly mixture forms.
2. Coat the fillets with flour and shake off the excess flour.
3. Next, dip the fillets in the egg.
4. Then coat the fillets with sesame seeds mixture generously.
5. Preheat the air fryer oven to 390 degrees F.
6. Air Frying. Line an Air fryer rack/basket with a piece of foil. Arrange the fillets into prepared basket.
7. Cook for about 14 minutes, flipping once after 10 minutes.

311.Panko-crusted Tilapia

Servings: 3
Cooking Time: 10 Minutes
Ingredients:
- 2 tsp. Italian seasoning
- 2 tsp. lemon pepper
- 1/3 C. panko breadcrumbs
- 1/3 C. egg whites
- 1/3 C. almond flour
- 3 tilapia fillets
- Olive oil

Directions:
1. Preparing the Ingredients. Place panko, egg whites, and flour into separate bowls. Mix lemon pepper and Italian seasoning in with breadcrumbs.
2. Pat tilapia fillets dry. Dredge in flour, then egg, then breadcrumb mixture.
3. Air Frying. Add to the Oven rack/basket and spray lightly with olive oil. Place the Rack on the middle-shelf of the air fryer oven.
4. Cook 10-11 minutes at 400 degrees, making sure to flip halfway through cooking.
- **Nutrition Info:** CALORIES: 256; FAT: 9G; PROTEIN:39G; SUGAR:5G

312.Fish Oregano Fingers

Servings:x
Cooking Time:x
Ingredients:
- ½ lb. firm white fish fillet cut into Oregano Fingers
- 1 tbsp. lemon juice
- 2 cups of dry breadcrumbs
- 1 cup oil for frying
- 1 ½ tbsp. ginger-garlic paste
- 3 tbsp. lemon juice
- 2 tsp salt
- 1 ½ tsp pepper powder

- 1 tsp red chili flakes or to taste
- 3 eggs
- 5 tbsp. corn flour
- 2 tsp tomato ketchup

Directions:
1. Rub a little lemon juice on the Oregano Fingers and set aside. Wash the fish after an hour and pat dry. Make the marinade and transfer the Oregano Fingers into the marinade. Leave them on a plate to dry for fifteen minutes. Now cover the Oregano Fingers with the crumbs and set aside to dry for fifteen minutes.
2. Pre heat the oven at 160 degrees Fahrenheit for 5 minutes or so. Keep the fish in the fry basket now and close it properly.
3. Let the Oregano Fingers cook at the same temperature for another 25 minutes. In between the cooking process, toss the fish once in a while to avoid burning the food. Serve either with tomato ketchup or chili sauce. Mint sauce also works well with the fish.

313. Miso White Fish Fillets

Servings: 2
Cooking Time: 10 Minutes
Ingredients:
- 2 cod fish fillets
- 2 tbsp brown sugar
- 2 tbsp miso
- 1 tbsp garlic, chopped

Directions:
1. Fit the oven with the rack in position 2.
2. Add all ingredients to the zip-lock bag and marinate fish in the refrigerator overnight.
3. Place marinated fish fillets in the air fryer basket then place an air fryer basket in the baking pan.
4. Place a baking pan on the oven rack. Set to air fry at 350 F for 10 minutes.
5. Serve and enjoy.
- **Nutrition Info:** Calories 9 Fat 0.1 g Carbohydrates 0.5 g Sugar 0.3 g Protein 1.5 g Cholesterol 3 mg

314. Crispy Salmon With Lemon-butter Sauce

Servings:x
Cooking Time:x
Ingredients:
- 4 (4-6-oz) salmon fillets, patted dry
- Salt and pepper, to taste
- 2 Tbsp olive oil
- 1 large garlic clove, minced
- 1/3 cup dry white wine
- 2 Tbsp fresh lemon juice
- 1 lemon zested

- 3 Tbsp unsalted butter, diced
- 2 Tbsp chopped fresh dill

Directions:
1. Place oven over medium heat.
2. Sprinkle salt and pepper on salmon fillets and add 1 Tbsp oil to the pan.
3. Add salmon flesh side down and cook 3-4 minutes. Flip the salmon and cook an additional 3 minutes on skin side. Transfer to a plate.
4. Wipe out oven and add remaining Tbsp olive oil over medium heat.
5. Add garlic and saute for 1 minute.
6. Pour in white wine and lemon juice. Stir for one minute.
7. Add lemon zest and continue stirring until slightly reduced.
8. Reduce heat to low and add cubed butter, stirring after each addition.
9. Sprinkle in fresh dill and stir all together.
10. Season with salt and pepper and pour sauce over salmon fillets.

315. Baked Halibut Steaks With Parsley

Servings: 4
Cooking Time: 10 Minutes
Ingredients:
- 1 pound (454 g) halibut steaks
- ¼ cup vegetable oil
- 2½ tablespoons Worcester sauce
- 2 tablespoons honey
- 2 tablespoons vermouth
- 1 tablespoon freshly squeezed lemon juice
- 1 tablespoon fresh parsley leaves, coarsely chopped
- Salt and pepper, to taste
- 1 teaspoon dried basil

Directions:
1. Put all the ingredients in a large mixing dish and gently stir until the fish is coated evenly. Transfer the fish to the baking pan.
2. Slide the baking pan into Rack Position 1, select Convection Bake, set temperature to 375ºF (190ºC), and set time to 10 minutes.
3. Flip the fish halfway through cooking time.
4. When cooking is complete, the fish should reach an internal temperature of at least 145ºF (63ºC) on a meat thermometer. Remove from the oven and let the fish cool for 5 minutes before serving.

316. Lemon Butter Shrimp

Servings: 4
Cooking Time: 12 Minutes
Ingredients:
- 1 1/4 lbs shrimp, peeled & deveined
- 2 tbsp fresh parsley, chopped
- 2 tbsp fresh lemon juice
- 1 tbsp garlic, minced

- 1/4 cup butter
- Pepper
- Salt

Directions:
1. Fit the oven with the rack in position
2. Add shrimp into the baking dish.
3. Melt butter in a pan over low heat. Add garlic and sauté for 30 seconds. Stir in lemon juice.
4. Pour melted butter mixture over shrimp. Season with pepper and salt.
5. Set to bake at 350 F for 17 minutes. After 5 minutes place the baking dish in the preheated oven.
6. Garnish with parsley and serve.
- **Nutrition Info:** Calories 276 Fat 14 g Carbohydrates 3.2 g Sugar 0.2 g Protein 32.7 g Cholesterol 329 mg

317.Tuna Lettuce Wraps

Servings:4
Cooking Time: 4 To 7 Minutes
Ingredients:
- 1 pound (454 g) fresh tuna steak, cut into 1-inch cubes
- 2 garlic cloves, minced
- 1 tablespoon grated fresh ginger
- ½ teaspoon toasted sesame oil
- 4 low-sodium whole-wheat tortillas
- 2 cups shredded romaine lettuce
- 1 red bell pepper, thinly sliced
- ¼ cup low-fat mayonnaise

Directions:
1. Combine the tuna cubes, garlic, ginger, and sesame oil in a medium bowl and toss until well coated. Allow to sit for 10 minutes.
2. When ready, place the tuna cubes in the air fryer basket.
3. Put the air fryer basket on the baking pan and slide into Rack Position 2, select Air Fry, set temperature to 390ºF (199ºC), and set time to 6 minutes.
4. When cooking is complete, the tuna cubes should be cooked through and golden brown. Remove the tuna cubes from the oven to a plate.
5. Make the wraps: Place the tortillas on a flat work surface and top each tortilla evenly with the cooked tuna, lettuce, bell pepper, and finish with the mayonnaise. Roll them up and serve immediately.

318.Lemon Tilapia

Servings:4
Cooking Time: 12 Minutes
Ingredients:
- 1 tablespoon olive oil
- 1 tablespoon lemon juice
- 1 teaspoon minced garlic

- ½ teaspoon chili powder
- 4 tilapia fillets

Directions:
1. Line the baking pan with parchment paper.
2. In a shallow bowl, stir together the olive oil, lemon juice, garlic, and chili powder to make a marinade. Put the tilapia fillets in the bowl, turning to coat evenly.
3. Place the fillets in the baking pan in a single layer.
4. Put the air fryer basket on the baking pan and slide into Rack Position 2, select Air Fry, set temperature to 375ºF (190ºC), and set time to 12 minutes.
5. When cooked, the fish will flake apart with a fork. Remove from the oven to a plate and serve hot.

319.Prawn French Cuisine Galette

Servings:x
Cooking Time:x
Ingredients:
- 2 tbsp. garam masala
- 1 lb. minced prawn
- 3 tsp ginger finely chopped
- 1-2 tbsp. fresh coriander leaves
- 2 or 3 green chilies finely chopped
- 1 ½ tbsp. lemon juice
- Salt and pepper to taste

Directions:
1. Mix the ingredients in a clean bowl.
2. Mold this mixture into round and flat French Cuisine Galettes.
3. Wet the French Cuisine Galettes slightly with water.
4. Pre heat the oven at 160 degrees Fahrenheit for 5 minutes. Place the French Cuisine Galettes in the fry basket and let them cook for another 25 minutes at the same temperature. Keep rolling them over to get a uniform cook. Serve either with mint sauce or ketchup.

320.Old Bay Tilapia Fillets

Servings: 4
Cooking Time: 15 Minutes
Ingredients:
- 1 pound tilapia fillets
- 1 tbsp old bay seasoning
- 2 tbsp canola oil
- 2 tbsp lemon pepper
- Salt to taste
- 2-3 butter buds

Directions:
1. Preheat your oven to 400 F on Bake function. Drizzle tilapia fillets with canola oil. In a bowl, mix salt, lemon pepper, butter buds, and seasoning; spread on the fish. Place the fillet on the basket and fit in the

baking tray. Cook for 10 minutes, flipping once until tender and crispy.

321.Bacon-wrapped Scallops

Servings:4
Cooking Time: 10 Minutes
Ingredients:
- 8 slices bacon, cut in half
- 16 sea scallops, patted dry
- Cooking spray
- Salt and freshly ground black pepper, to taste
- 16 toothpicks, soaked in water for at least 30 minutes

Directions:
1. On a clean work surface, wrap half of a slice of bacon around each scallop and secure with a toothpick.
2. Lay the bacon-wrapped scallops in the air fryer basket in a single layer.
3. Spritz the scallops with cooking spray and sprinkle the salt and pepper to season.
4. Put the air fryer basket on the baking pan and slide into Rack Position 2, select Air Fry, set temperature to 370ºF (188ºC), and set time to 10 minutes.
5. Flip the scallops halfway through the cooking time.
6. When cooking is complete, the bacon should be cooked through and the scallops should be firm. Remove the scallops from the oven to a plate Serve warm.

322.Quick Paella

Servings: 4
Cooking Time: 15 Minutes
Ingredients:
- 1 (10-ounce) package frozen cooked rice, thawed
- 1 (6-ounce) jar artichoke hearts, drained and chopped
- ¼ cup vegetable broth
- ½ teaspoon turmeric
- ½ teaspoon dried thyme
- 1 cup frozen cooked small shrimp
- ½ cup frozen baby peas
- 1 tomato, diced

Directions:
1. Preparing the Ingredients. In a 6-by-6-by-2-inch pan, combine the rice, artichoke hearts, vegetable broth, turmeric, and thyme, and stir gently.
2. Air Frying. Place in the air fryer oven and bake for 8 to 9 minutes or until the rice is hot. Remove from the air fryer oven and gently stir in the shrimp, peas, and tomato. Cook for 5 to 8 minutes or until the shrimp and peas are hot and the paella is bubbling.

- **Nutrition Info:** CALORIES: 345; FAT: 1G; PROTEIN:18G; FIBER:4G

323.Asian-inspired Swordfish Steaks

Servings:4
Cooking Time: 8 Minutes
Ingredients:
- 4 (4-ounce / 113-g) swordfish steaks
- ½ teaspoon toasted sesame oil
- 1 jalapeño pepper, finely minced
- 2 garlic cloves, grated
- 2 tablespoons freshly squeezed lemon juice
- 1 tablespoon grated fresh ginger
- ½ teaspoon Chinese five-spice powder
- ⅛ teaspoon freshly ground black pepper

Directions:
1. On a clean work surface, place the swordfish steaks and brush both sides of the fish with the sesame oil.
2. Combine the jalapeño, garlic, lemon juice, ginger, five-spice powder, and black pepper in a small bowl and stir to mix well. Rub the mixture all over the fish until completely coated. Allow to sit for 10 minutes.
3. When ready, arrange the swordfish steaks in the air fryer basket.
4. Put the air fryer basket on the baking pan and slide into Rack Position 2, select Air Fry, set temperature to 380ºF (193ºC), and set time to 8 minutes.
5. Flip the steaks halfway through.
6. When cooking is complete, remove from the oven and cool for 5 minutes before serving.

324.Mustard-crusted Sole Fillets

Servings:4
Cooking Time: 10 Minutes
Ingredients:
- 5 teaspoons low-sodium yellow mustard
- 1 tablespoon freshly squeezed lemon juice
- 4 (3.5-ounce / 99-g) sole fillets
- 2 teaspoons olive oil
- ½ teaspoon dried marjoram
- ½ teaspoon dried thyme
- ⅛ teaspoon freshly ground black pepper
- 1 slice low-sodium whole-wheat bread, crumbled

Directions:
1. Whisk together the mustard and lemon juice in a small bowl until thoroughly mixed and smooth. Spread the mixture evenly over the sole fillets, then transfer the fillets to the baking pan.
2. In a separate bowl, combine the olive oil, marjoram, thyme, black pepper, and bread crumbs and stir to mix well. Gently but firmly press the mixture onto the top of fillets, coating them completely.

3. Slide the baking pan into Rack Position 1, select Convection Bake, set temperature to 320ºF (160ºC), and set time to 10 minutes.
4. When cooking is complete, the fish should reach an internal temperature of 145ºF (63ºC) on a meat thermometer. Remove from the oven and serve on a plate.

325.Breaded Seafood

Servings:4
Cooking Time: 15 Minutes
Ingredients:
- 1 lb scallops, mussels, fish fillets, prawns, shrimp
- 2 eggs, lightly beaten
- Salt and black pepper to taste
- 1 cup breadcrumbs mixed with zest of 1 lemon

Directions:
1. Dip the seafood pieces into the eggs and season with salt and black pepper. Coat in the crumbs and spray with cooking spray. Arrange them on the frying basket and press Start. Cook for 10 minutes at 400 F on AirFry function. Serve with lemon wedges.

326.Tasty Parmesan Shrimp

Servings: 4
Cooking Time: 10 Minutes
Ingredients:
- 1 lb shrimp, peeled and deveined
- 1/4 cup parmesan cheese, grated
- 4 garlic cloves, minced
- 1 tbsp olive oil
- 1/4 tsp oregano
- 1/2 tsp pepper
- 1/2 tsp onion powder
- 1/2 tsp basil

Directions:
1. Fit the oven with the rack in position 2.
2. Add all ingredients into the large bowl and toss well.
3. Add shrimp to the air fryer basket then place an air fryer basket in the baking pan.
4. Place a baking pan on the oven rack. Set to air fry at 350 F for 10 minutes.
5. Serve and enjoy.
- **Nutrition Info:** Calories 189 Fat 6.7 g Carbohydrates 3.4 g Sugar 0.1 g Protein 27.9 g Cholesterol 243 mg

327.Spinach & Tuna Balls With Ricotta

Servings:4
Cooking Time: 20 Minutes
Ingredients:
- 14 oz store-bought crescent dough
- ½ cup spinach, steamed
- 1 cup ricotta cheese, crumbled
- ¼ tsp garlic powder
- 1 tsp fresh oregano, chopped
- ½ cup canned tuna, drained

Directions:
1. Preheat on AirFry function to 350 F. Roll the dough onto a lightly floured flat surface. Combine the ricotta cheese, spinach, tuna, oregano, salt, and garlic powder together in a bowl.
2. Cut the dough into 4 equal pieces. Divide the mixture between the dough pieces. Make sure to place the filling in the center. Fold the dough and secure with a fork. Place onto a lined baking dish and press Start. Cook for 12 minutes until lightly browned. Serve.

328.Lemony Tuna

Servings: 4
Cooking Time: 10 Minutes
Ingredients:
- 2 (6-ounce) cans water packed plain tuna
- 2 teaspoons Dijon mustard
- ½ cup breadcrumbs
- 1 tablespoon fresh lime juice
- 2 tablespoons fresh parsley, chopped
- 1 egg
- Chefman of hot sauce
- 3 tablespoons canola oil
- Salt and freshly ground black pepper, to taste

Directions:
1. Preparing the Ingredients. Drain most of the liquid from the canned tuna.
2. In a bowl, add the fish, mustard, crumbs, citrus juice, parsley, and hot sauce and mix till well combined. Add a little canola oil if it seems too dry. Add egg, salt and stir to combine. Make the patties from tuna mixture. Refrigerate the tuna patties for about 2 hours.
3. Air Frying. Preheat the air fryer oven to 355 degrees F. Cook for about 10-12 minutes.

329.Crispy Coated Scallops

Servings: 4
Cooking Time: 10 Minutes
Ingredients:
- Nonstick cooking spray
- 1 lb. sea scallops, patted dry
- 1 teaspoon onion powder
- ½ tsp pepper
- 1 egg
- 1 tbsp. water
- ¼ cup Italian bread crumbs
- Paprika
- 1 tbsp. fresh lemon juice

Directions:

1. Lightly spray fryer basket with cooking spray. Place baking pan in position 2 of the oven.
2. Sprinkle scallops with onion powder and pepper.
3. In a shallow dish, whisk together egg and water.
4. Place bread crumbs in a separate shallow dish.
5. Dip scallops in egg then bread crumbs coating them lightly. Place in fryer basket and lightly spray with cooking spray. Sprinkle with paprika.
6. Place the basket on the baking pan and set oven to air fryer on 400°F. Bake 10-12 minutes until scallops are firm on the inside and golden brown on the outside. Drizzle with lemon juice and serve.
- **Nutrition Info:** Calories 122, Total Fat 2g, Saturated Fat 1g, Total Carbs 10g, Net Carbs 9g, Protein 16g, Sugar 1g, Fiber 1g, Sodium 563mg, Potassium 282mg, Phosphorus 420mg

330.Baked Buttery Shrimp

Servings: 4
Cooking Time: 15 Minutes
Ingredients:
- 1 lb shrimp, peel & deveined
- 2 tsp garlic powder
- 2 tsp dry mustard
- 2 tsp cumin
- 2 tsp paprika
- 2 tsp black pepper
- 4 tsp cayenne pepper
- 1/2 cup butter, melted
- 2 tsp onion powder
- 1 tsp dried oregano
- 1 tsp dried thyme
- 3 tsp salt

Directions:
1. Fit the oven with the rack in position
2. Add shrimp, butter, and remaining ingredients into the mixing bowl and toss well.
3. Transfer shrimp mixture into the baking pan.
4. Set to bake at 400 F for 20 minutes. After 5 minutes place the baking pan in the preheated oven.
5. Serve and enjoy.
- **Nutrition Info:** Calories 372 Fat 26.2 g Carbohydrates 7.5 g Sugar 1.3 g Protein 27.6 g Cholesterol 300 mg

331.Paprika Shrimp

Servings:4
Cooking Time: 10 Minutes
Ingredients:

- 1 pound (454 g) tiger shrimp
- 2 tablespoons olive oil
- ½ tablespoon old bay seasoning
- ¼ tablespoon smoked paprika
- ¼ teaspoon cayenne pepper
- A pinch of sea salt

Directions:
1. Toss all the ingredients in a large bowl until the shrimp are evenly coated.
2. Arrange the shrimp in the air fryer basket.
3. Put the air fryer basket on the baking pan and slide into Rack Position 2, select Air Fry, set temperature to 380ºF (193ºC), and set time to 10 minutes.
4. When cooking is complete, the shrimp should be pink and cooked through. Remove from the oven and serve hot.

332.Fish And Chips

Servings: 4
Cooking Time: 20 Minutes
Ingredients:
- 4 (4-ounce) fish fillets
- Pinch salt
- Freshly ground black pepper
- ½ teaspoon dried thyme
- 1 egg white
- ¾ cup crushed potato chips
- 2 tablespoons olive oil, divided
- 1 russet potatoes, peeled and cut into strips

Directions:
1. Preparing the Ingredients. Pat the fish fillets dry and sprinkle with salt, pepper, and thyme. Set aside.
2. In a shallow bowl, beat the egg white until foamy. In another bowl, combine the potato chips and 1 tablespoon of olive oil and mix until combined.
3. Dip the fish fillets into the egg white, then into the crushed potato chip mixture to coat.
4. Toss the fresh potato strips with the remaining 1 tablespoon olive oil.
5. Air Frying. Use your separator to divide the Oven rack/basket in half, then fry the chips and fish. The chips will take about 20 minutes; the fish will take about 10 to 12 minutes to cook.
- **Nutrition Info:** CALORIES: 374; FAT:16G; PROTEIN:30G; FIBER:4G

333.Simple Salmon Patties

Servings: 2
Cooking Time: 7 Minutes
Ingredients:
- 8 oz salmon fillet, minced
- 1 egg, lightly beaten
- 1/4 tsp garlic powder
- 1/4 tsp onion powder

- 1/8 tsp paprika
- 2 tbsp breadcrumbs
- Pepper
- Salt

Directions:
1. Fit the oven with the rack in position 2.
2. Add all ingredients into the bowl and mix until well combined.
3. Make patties from mixture and place in the air fryer basket then place an air fryer basket in the baking pan.
4. Place a baking pan on the oven rack. Set to air fry at 390 F for 7 minutes.
5. Serve and enjoy.
- **Nutrition Info:** Calories 211 Fat 9.6 g Carbohydrates 5.6 g Sugar 0.8 g Protein 25.8 g Cholesterol 132 mg

334.Easy Shrimp Fajitas

Servings: 10
Cooking Time: 20 Minutes
Ingredients:
- 1 lb shrimp
- 1 tbsp olive oil
- 2 bell peppers, diced
- 2 tbsp taco seasoning
- 1/2 cup onion, diced

Directions:
1. Fit the oven with the rack in position 2.
2. Add shrimp and remaining ingredients into the bowl and toss well.
3. Add shrimp mixture to the air fryer basket then place an air fryer basket in baking pan.
4. Place a baking pan on the oven rack. Set to air fry at 390 F for 20 minutes.
5. Serve and enjoy.
- **Nutrition Info:** Calories 76 Fat 2.2 g Carbohydrates 3 g Sugar 1.4 g Protein 10.6 g Cholesterol 96 mg

335.Smoked Paprika Tiger Shrimp

Servings:4
Cooking Time: 10 Minutes
Ingredients:
- 1 lb tiger shrimp
- 2 tbsp olive oil
- ¼ tbsp garlic powder
- 1 tbsp smoked paprika
- 2 tbsp fresh parsley, chopped
- Sea salt to taste

Directions:
1. Preheat on AirFry function to 380 F. Mix garlic powder, smoked paprika, salt, parsley, and olive oil in a large bowl. Add in the shrimp and toss to coat. Place the shrimp in the frying basket press Start. Fry for 6-7 minutes. Serve with salad.

336.Golden Beer-battered Cod

Servings:4
Cooking Time: 15 Minutes
Ingredients:
- 2 eggs
- 1 cup malty beer
- 1 cup all-purpose flour
- ½ cup cornstarch
- 1 teaspoon garlic powder
- Salt and pepper, to taste
- 4 (4-ounce / 113-g) cod fillets
- Cooking spray

Directions:
1. In a shallow bowl, beat together the eggs with the beer. In another shallow bowl, thoroughly combine the flour and cornstarch. Sprinkle with the garlic powder, salt, and pepper.
2. Dredge each cod fillet in the flour mixture, then in the egg mixture. Dip each piece of fish in the flour mixture a second time.
3. Spritz the air fryer basket with cooking spray. Arrange the cod fillets in the pan in a single layer.
4. Put the air fryer basket on the baking pan and slide into Rack Position 2, select Air Fry, set temperature to 400ºF (205ºC), and set time to 15 minutes.
5. Flip the fillets halfway through the cooking time.
6. When cooking is complete, the cod should reach an internal temperature of 145ºF (63ºC) on a meat thermometer and the outside should be crispy. Let the fish cool for 5 minutes and serve.

337.Rosemary Garlic Shrimp

Servings: 4
Cooking Time: 10 Minutes
Ingredients:
- 1 lb shrimp, peeled and deveined
- 2 garlic cloves, minced
- 1/2 tbsp fresh rosemary, chopped
- 1 tbsp olive oil
- Pepper
- Salt

Directions:
1. Fit the oven with the rack in position
2. Add shrimp and remaining ingredients in a large bowl and toss well.
3. Pour shrimp mixture into the baking dish.
4. Set to bake at 400 F for 15 minutes. After 5 minutes place the baking dish in the preheated oven.
5. Serve and enjoy.
- **Nutrition Info:** Calories 168 Fat 5.5 g Carbohydrates 2.5 g Sugar 0 g Protein 26 g Cholesterol 239 mg

338. Baked Flounder Fillets

Servings: 2
Cooking Time: 12 Minutes
Ingredients:
- 2 flounder fillets, patted dry
- 1 egg
- ½ teaspoon Worcestershire sauce
- ¼ cup almond flour
- ¼ cup coconut flour
- ½ teaspoon coarse sea salt
- ½ teaspoon lemon pepper
- ¼ teaspoon chili powder
- Cooking spray

Directions:
1. In a shallow bowl, beat together the egg with Worcestershire sauce until well incorporated.
2. In another bowl, thoroughly combine the almond flour, coconut flour, sea salt, lemon pepper, and chili powder.
3. Dredge the fillets in the egg mixture, shaking off any excess, then roll in the flour mixture to coat well.
4. Spritz the baking pan with cooking spray. Place the fillets in the pan.
5. Slide the baking pan into Rack Position 1, select Convection Bake, set temperature to 390ºF (199ºC), and set time to 12 minutes.
6. After 7 minutes, remove from the oven and flip the fillets and spray with cooking spray. Return the pan to the oven and continue cooking for 5 minutes, or until the fish is flaky.
7. When cooking is complete, remove from the oven and serve warm.

339. Baked Pesto Salmon

Servings: 4
Cooking Time: 15 Minutes
Ingredients:
- 4 salmon fillets
- 1/3 cup parmesan cheese, grated
- 1/3 cup breadcrumbs
- 6 tbsp pesto

Directions:
1. Fit the oven with the rack in position
2. Place fish fillets into the baking dish.
3. Pour pesto over fish fillets.
4. Mix together breadcrumbs and parmesan cheese and sprinkle over fish.
5. Set to bake at 325 F for 20 minutes. After 5 minutes place the baking dish in the preheated oven.
6. Serve and enjoy.
- **Nutrition Info:** Calories 396 Fat 22.8 g Carbohydrates 8.3 g Sugar 2.1 g Protein 40.4 g Cholesterol 89 mg

340. Old Bay Crab Cakes

Servings: 4
Cooking Time: 20 Minutes
Ingredients:
- 2 slices dried bread, crusts removed
- Small amount of milk
- 1 tablespoon mayonnaise
- 1 tablespoon Worcestershire sauce
- 1 tablespoon baking powder
- 1 tablespoon parsley flakes
- 1 teaspoon Old Bay® Seasoning
- 1/4 teaspoon salt
- 1 egg
- 1 pound lump crabmeat

Directions:
1. Preparing the Ingredients. Crush your bread over a large bowl until it is broken down into small pieces. Add milk and stir until bread crumbs are moistened. Mix in mayo and Worcestershire sauce. Add remaining ingredients and mix well. Shape into 4 patties.
2. Air Frying. Cook at 360 degrees for 20 minutes, flip half way through.
- **Nutrition Info:** CALORIES: 165; CARBS:5.8; FAT: 4.5G; PROTEIN:24G; FIBER:0G

341. Roasted Salmon With Asparagus

Servings: 4
Cooking Time: 15 Minutes
Ingredients:
- 4 (6-ounce / 170 g) salmon fillets, patted dry
- 1 teaspoon kosher salt, divided
- 1 tablespoon honey
- 2 tablespoons unsalted butter, melted
- 2 teaspoons Dijon mustard
- 2 pounds (907 g) asparagus, trimmed
- Lemon wedges, for serving

Directions:
1. Season both sides of the salmon fillets with ½ teaspoon of kosher salt.
2. Whisk together the honey, 1 tablespoon of butter, and mustard in a small bowl. Set aside.
3. Arrange the asparagus in the baking pan. Drizzle the remaining 1 tablespoon of butter all over and season with the remaining ½ teaspoon of salt, tossing to coat. Move the asparagus to the outside of the pan.
4. Put the salmon fillets in the pan, skin-side down. Brush the fillets generously with the honey mixture.
5. Slide the baking pan into Rack Position 2, select Roast, set temperature to 375ºF (190ºC), and set time to 15 minutes.
6. Toss the asparagus once halfway through the cooking time.

7. When done, transfer the salmon fillets and asparagus to a plate. Serve warm with a squeeze of lemon juice.

342.Delicious Shrimp Casserole

Servings: 10
Cooking Time: 30 Minutes
Ingredients:
- 1 lb shrimp, peeled & tail off
- 2 tsp onion powder
- 2 tsp old bay seasoning
- 2 cups cheddar cheese, shredded
- 10.5 oz can cream of mushroom soup
- 12 oz long-grain rice
- 1 tsp salt

Directions:

1. Fit the oven with the rack in position
2. Cook rice according to the packet instructions.
3. Add shrimp into the boiling water and cook for 4 minutes or until cooked. Drain shrimp.
4. In a bowl, mix rice, shrimp, and remaining ingredients and pour into the greased 13*9-inch casserole dish.
5. Set to bake at 350 F for 35 minutes. After 5 minutes place the casserole dish in the preheated oven.
6. Serve and enjoy.
- **Nutrition Info:** Calories 286 Fat 9 g Carbohydrates 31 g Sugar 1 g Protein 18.8 g Cholesterol 120 mg

MEATLESS RECIPES

343.Roasted Carrots

Servings: 4
Cooking Time: 15 Minutes
Ingredients:
- 20 oz carrots, julienned
- 1 tbsp olive oil
- 1 tsp cumin seeds
- 2 tbsp fresh cilantro, chopped

Directions:
1. In a bowl, mix olive oil, carrots, and cumin seeds; stir to coat. Place the carrots in a baking tray and cook in your on Bake function at 300 F for 10 minutes. Scatter fresh coriander over the carrots and serve.

344.Awesome Sweet Potato Fries

Servings: 4
Cooking Time: 30 Minutes
Ingredients:
- ½ tsp salt
- ½ tsp garlic powder
- ½ tsp chili powder
- ¼ tsp cumin
- 3 tbsp olive oil
- 3 sweet potatoes, cut into thick strips

Directions:
1. In a bowl, mix salt, garlic powder, chili, and cumin, and olive oil. Coat the strips well in this mixture and arrange them in the basket without overcrowding. Fit in the baking tray and cook for 20 minutes at 380 F on Air Fry function or until crispy. Serve.

345.Grandma´s Ratatouille

Servings:2
Cooking Time: 30 Minutes
Ingredients:
- 1 tbsp olive oil
- 3 Roma tomatoes, thinly sliced
- 2 garlic cloves, minced
- 1 zucchini, thinly sliced
- 2 yellow bell peppers, sliced
- 1 tbsp vinegar
- 2 tbsp herbs de Provence
- Salt and black pepper to taste

Directions:
1. Preheat on AirFry function to 390 F. Place all ingredients in a bowl. Season with salt and pepper and stir to coat. Arrange the vegetable on a baking dish and place in the oven. Cook for 15 minutes, shaking occasionally. Let sit for 5 more minutes after the timer goes off.

346.Stuffed Mushrooms

Servings: 12
Cooking Time: 8 Minutes
Ingredients:
- 2 Rashers Bacon, Diced
- ½ Onion, Diced
- ½ Bell Pepper, Diced
- 1 Small Carrot, Diced
- 24 Medium Size Mushrooms (Separate the caps & stalks)
- 1 cup Shredded Cheddar Plus Extra for the Top
- ½ cup Sour Cream

Directions:
1. Preparing the Ingredients. Chop the mushrooms stalks finely and fry them up with the bacon, onion, pepper and carrot at 350 ° for 8 minutes.
2. When the veggies are fairly tender, stir in the sour cream & the cheese. Keep on the heat until the cheese has melted and everything is mixed nicely.
3. Now grab the mushroom caps and heap a plop of filling on each one.
4. Place in the fryer basket and top with a little extra cheese.

347.Bottle Gourd Flat Cakes

Servings:x
Cooking Time:x
Ingredients:
- 2 or 3 green chilies finely chopped
- 1 ½ tbsp. lemon juice
- Salt and pepper to taste
- 2 tbsp. garam masala
- 2 cups sliced bottle gourd
- 3 tsp. ginger finely chopped
- 1-2 tbsp. fresh coriander leaves

Directions:
1. Mix the ingredients in a clean bowl and add water to it. Make sure that the paste is not too watery but is enough to apply on the bottle gourd slices. Pre heat the oven at 160 degrees Fahrenheit for 5 minutes.
2. Place the French Cuisine Galettes in the fry basket and let them cook for another 25 minutes at the same temperature. Keep rolling them over to get a uniform cook. Serve either with mint sauce or ketchup.

348.Crispy Fried Okra With Chili

Servings:4
Cooking Time: 10 Minutes
Ingredients:
- 3 tablespoons sour cream
- 2 tablespoons flour
- 2 tablespoons semolina
- ½ teaspoon red chili powder
- Salt and black pepper, to taste
- 1 pound (454 g) okra, halved
- Cooking spray

Directions:
1. Spray the air fryer basket with cooking spray. Set aside.
2. In a shallow bowl, place the sour cream. In another shallow bowl, thoroughly combine the flour, semolina, red chili powder, salt, and pepper.
3. Dredge the okra in the sour cream, then roll in the flour mixture until evenly coated. Transfer the okra to the air fryer basket.
4. Put the air fryer basket on the baking pan and slide into Rack Position 2, select Air Fry, set temperature to 400ºF (205ºC), and set time to 10 minutes.
5. Flip the okra halfway through the cooking time.
6. When cooking is complete, the okra should be golden brown and crispy. Remove from the oven and cool for 5 minutes before serving.

349.Cheesy Spinach Toasties

Servings:x
Cooking Time:x
Ingredients:
- 1 tsp. coarsely crushed green chilies
- 2 tbsp. grated pizza cheese
- 1 cup milk
- 2 toasted bread slices cut into triangles
- 1 tbsp. butter
- 1 tbsp. all-purpose flour
- 1 small onion finely chopped
- 1-2 flakes garlic finely chopped
- Half a bunch of spinach that has been boiled and crushed (does not have to
- be crushed finely)
- 1 tbsp. fresh cream
- Some salt and pepper to taste

Directions:
1. Take a pan and melt some butter in it. Also add some onions and garlic.
2. Now keep roasting them in the butter until the onions are caramelized or attain a golden-brown color.
3. Into this pan add the required amount of all-purpose flour. Continue to roast for 3 minutes or so. Add milk and keep stirring until you bring it to a boil.
4. Add green chilies, cream, spinach and seasoning. Mix the ingredients properly and let it cook until the mixture thickens. Toast some bread. Apply the paste made in the previous step on the bread.
5. Sprinkle some grated cheese on top of the paste.
6. Pre heat the oven at 290 Fahrenheit for around 4 minutes. Put the toasts in the Fry basket and let it continue to cook for

another 10 minutes at the same temperature.

350.Cheese Stuffed Green Peppers With Tomato Sauce

Servings:4
Cooking Time: 35 Minutes
Ingredients:
- 2 cans green chili peppers
- 1 cup cheddar cheese, shredded
- 1 cup Monterey Jack cheese, shredded
- 2 tbsp all-purpose flour
- 2 large eggs, beaten
- ½ cup milk
- 1 can tomato sauce

Directions:
1. Preheat on AirFry function to 380 F. Spray a baking dish with cooking spray. Take half of the chilies and arrange them in the baking dish. Top with half of the cheese and cover with the remaining chilies. In a medium bowl, combine eggs, milk, and flour and pour over the chilies.
2. Press Start and cook for 20 minutes. Remove the chilies and pour the tomato sauce over them; cook for 15 more minutes. Top with the remaining cheese and serve.

351.Spicy Kung Pao Tofu

Servings:4
Cooking Time: 10 Minutes
Ingredients:
- $^1/_3$ cup Asian-Style sauce
- 1 teaspoon cornstarch
- ½ teaspoon red pepper flakes, or more to taste
- 1 pound (454 g) firm or extra-firm tofu, cut into 1-inch cubes
- 1 small carrot, peeled and cut into ¼-inch-thick coins
- 1 small green bell pepper, cut into bite-size pieces
- 3 scallions, sliced, whites and green parts separated
- 3 tablespoons roasted unsalted peanuts

Directions:
1. In a large bowl, whisk together the sauce, cornstarch, and red pepper flakes. Fold in the tofu, carrot, pepper, and the white parts of the scallions and toss to coat. Spread the mixture evenly in the baking pan.
2. Slide the baking pan into Rack Position 2, select Roast, set temperature to 375ºF (190ºC), and set time to 10 minutes.
3. Stir the ingredients once halfway through the cooking time.
4. When done, remove from the oven. Serve sprinkled with the peanuts and scallion greens.

352.Pizza

Servings:x
Cooking Time:x
Ingredients:
- 2 tomatoes that have been deseeded and chopped
- 1 tbsp. (optional) mushrooms/corns
- 2 tsp. pizza seasoning
- Some cottage cheese that has been cut into small cubes (optional)
- One pizza base
- Grated pizza cheese (mozzarella cheese preferably) for topping
- Use cooking oil for brushing and topping purposes
- ingredients for topping:
- 2 onions chopped
- 2 capsicums chopped

Directions:
1. Put the pizza base in a pre-heated oven for around 5 minutes. (Pre heated to 340 Fahrenheit). Take out the base.
2. Pour some pizza sauce on top of the base at the center. Using a spoon spread the sauce over the base making sure that you leave some gap around the circumference. Grate some mozzarella cheese and sprinkle it over the sauce layer. Take all the vegetables mentioned in the ingredient list above and mix them in a bowl.
3. Add some oil and seasoning. Also add some salt and pepper according to taste. Mix them properly. Put this topping over the layer of cheese on the pizza. Now sprinkle some more grated cheese and pizza seasoning on top of this layer.
4. Pre heat the oven at 250 Fahrenheit for around 5 minutes. Open the fry basket and place the pizza inside. Close the basket and keep the fryer at 170 degrees for another 10 minutes. If you feel that it is undercooked you may put it at the same temperature for another 2 minutes or so.

353.Cabbage Fritters(2)

Servings:x
Cooking Time:x
Ingredients:
- 1 ½ tsp. salt
- 3 tsp. lemon juice
- 2 tsp. garam masala
- 3 eggs
- 2 ½ tbsp. white sesame seeds
- 10 leaves cabbage
- 3 onions chopped
- 5 green chilies-roughly chopped
- 1 ½ tbsp. ginger paste
- 1 ½ tsp. garlic paste

Directions:

1. Grind the ingredients except for the egg and form a smooth paste. Coat the leaves in the paste. Now, beat the eggs and add a little salt to it.
2. Dip the coated leaves in the egg mixture and then transfer to the sesame seeds and coat the florets well. Place the vegetables on a stick.
3. Pre heat the oven at 160 degrees Fahrenheit for around 5 minutes. Place the sticks in the basket and let them cook for another 25 minutes at the same temperature. Turn the sticks over in between the cooking process to get a uniform cook.

354.Baked Turnip And Zucchini

Servings:4
Cooking Time: 18 Minutes
Ingredients:
- 3 turnips, sliced
- 1 large zucchini, sliced
- 1 large red onion, cut into rings
- 2 cloves garlic, crushed
- 1 tablespoon olive oil
- Salt and black pepper, to taste

Directions:
1. Put the turnips, zucchini, red onion, and garlic in the baking pan. Drizzle the olive oil over the top and sprinkle with the salt and pepper.
2. Slide the baking pan into Rack Position 1, select Convection Bake, set temperature to 330ºF (166ºC), and set time to 18 minutes.
3. When cooking is complete, the vegetables should be tender. Remove from the oven and serve on a plate.

355.Broccoli Momo's Recipe

Servings:x
Cooking Time:x
Ingredients:
- 2 tbsp. oil
- 2 tsp. ginger-garlic paste
- 2 tsp. soya sauce
- 2 tsp. vinegar
- 1 ½ cup all-purpose flour
- ½ tsp. salt
- 5 tbsp. water
- 2 cups grated broccoli

Directions:
1. Squeeze the dough and cover it with plastic wrap and set aside. Next, cook the ingredients for the filling and try to ensure that the broccoli is covered well with the sauce.
2. Roll the dough and cut it into a square. Place the filling in the center. Now, wrap the

dough to cover the filling and pinch the edges together.

3. Pre heat the oven at 200° F for 5 minutes. Place the gnocchi's in the fry basket and close it. Let them cook at the same temperature for another 20 minutes. Recommended sides are chili sauce or ketchup.

356.Parmesan Coated Green Beans

Servings:4
Cooking Time: 20 Minutes
Ingredients:
- 1 cup panko breadcrumbs
- 2 whole eggs, beaten
- ½ cup Parmesan cheese, grated
- ½ cup flour
- 1 tsp cayenne pepper powder
- 1 ½ pounds green beans
- Salt to taste

Directions:
1. Preheat on AirFry function to 380 F. In a bowl, mix breadcrumbs, Parmesan cheese, cayenne pepper powder, salt, and pepper. Flour the green beans and dip them in eggs. Dredge beans in the Parmesan-panko mix. Place in the cooking basket and cook for 15 minutes Serve.

357.Fenugreek French Cuisine Galette

Servings:x
Cooking Time:x
Ingredients:
- 2 or 3 green chilies finely chopped
- 1 ½ tbsp. lemon juice
- Salt and pepper to taste
- 2 cups fenugreek
- 2 medium potatoes boiled and mashed
- 3 tsp. ginger finely chopped
- 1-2 tbsp. fresh coriander leaves

Directions:
1. Mix the ingredients in a clean bowl.
2. Mold this mixture into round and flat French Cuisine Galettes.
3. Wet the French Cuisine Galettes slightly with water.
4. Pre heat the oven at 160 degrees Fahrenheit for 5 minutes. Place the French Cuisine Galettes in the fry basket and let them cook for another 25 minutes at the same temperature. Keep rolling them over to get a uniform cook. Serve either with mint sauce or ketchup.

358.Cream Cheese Stuffed Bell Peppers

Servings:2
Cooking Time: 15 Minutes
Ingredients:
- 2 bell peppers, tops and seeds removed

- Salt and pepper, to taste
- $^2/_3$ cup cream cheese
- 2 tablespoons mayonnaise
- 1 tablespoon chopped fresh celery stalks
- Cooking spray

Directions:
1. Spritz the air fryer basket with cooking spray.
2. Place the peppers in the air fryer basket.
3. Put the air fryer basket on the baking pan and slide into Rack Position 2, select Roast, set temperature to 400ºF (205ºC) and set time to 10 minutes.
4. Flip the peppers halfway through.
5. When cooking is complete, the peppers should be crisp-tender.
6. Remove from the oven to a plate and season with salt and pepper.
7. Mix the cream cheese, mayo, and celery in a small bowl and stir to incorporate. Evenly stuff the roasted peppers with the cream cheese mixture with a spoon. Serve immediately.

359.Roasted Vegetable Mélange With Herbs

Servings:4
Cooking Time: 16 Minutes
Ingredients:
- 1 (8-ounce / 227-g) package sliced mushrooms
- 1 yellow summer squash, sliced
- 1 red bell pepper, sliced
- 3 cloves garlic, sliced
- 1 tablespoon olive oil
- ½ teaspoon dried basil
- ½ teaspoon dried thyme
- ½ teaspoon dried tarragon

Directions:
1. Toss the mushrooms, squash, and bell pepper with the garlic and olive oil in a large bowl until well coated. Mix in the basil, thyme, and tarragon and toss again.
2. Spread the vegetables evenly in the air fryer basket.
3. Put the air fryer basket on the baking pan and slide into Rack Position 2, select Roast, set temperature to 350ºF (180ºC), and set time to 16 minutes.
4. When cooking is complete, the vegetables should be fork-tender. Remove from the oven and cool for 5 minutes before serving.

360.Roasted Butternut Squash With Maple Syrup

Servings:4
Cooking Time: 30 Minutes
Ingredients:
- 1 lb butternut squash

- 1 tsp dried rosemary
- 2 tbsp maple syrup
- Salt to taste

Directions:
1. Place the squash on a cutting board and peel. Cut in half and remove the seeds and pulp. Slice into wedges and season with salt. Spray with cooking spray and sprinkle with rosemary.
2. Preheat on AirFry function to 350 F. Transfer the wedges to the greased basket without overlapping. Press Start and cook for 20 minutes. Serve drizzled with maple syrup.

361.Caramelized Eggplant With Yogurt Sauce

Servings:2
Cooking Time: 15 Minutes
Ingredients:
- 1 medium eggplant, quartered and cut crosswise into ½-inch-thick slices
- 2 tablespoons vegetable oil
- Kosher salt and freshly ground black pepper, to taste
- ½ cup plain yogurt (not Greek)
- 2 tablespoons harissa paste
- 1 garlic clove, grated
- 2 teaspoons honey

Directions:
1. Toss the eggplant slices with the vegetable oil, salt, and pepper in a large bowl until well coated.
2. Lay the eggplant slices in the air fryer basket.
3. Put the air fryer basket on the baking pan and slide into Rack Position 2, select Air Fry, set temperature to 400ºF (205ºC), and set time to 15 minutes.
4. Stir the slices two to three times during cooking.
5. Meanwhile, make the yogurt sauce by whisking together the yogurt, harissa paste, and garlic in a small bowl.
6. When cooking is complete, the eggplant slices should be golden brown. Spread the yogurt sauce on a platter, and pile the eggplant slices over the top. Serve drizzled with the honey.

362.Cheese-walnut Stuffed Mushrooms

Servings:4
Cooking Time: 10 Minutes
Ingredients:
- 4 large portobello mushrooms
- 1 tablespoon canola oil
- ½ cup shredded Mozzarella cheese
- $^1/_3$ cup minced walnuts
- 2 tablespoons chopped fresh parsley

- Cooking spray

Directions:
1. Spritz the air fryer basket with cooking spray.
2. On a clean work surface, remove the mushroom stems. Scoop out the gills with a spoon and discard. Coat the mushrooms with canola oil. Top each mushroom evenly with the shredded Mozzarella cheese, followed by the minced walnuts.
3. Arrange the mushrooms in the basket.
4. Put the air fryer basket on the baking pan and slide into Rack Position 2, select Roast, set temperature to 350ºF (180ºC) and set time to 10 minutes.
5. When cooking is complete, the mushroom should be golden brown.
6. Transfer the mushrooms to a plate and sprinkle the parsley on top for garnish before serving.

363.Cottage Cheese Spicy Lemon Kebab

Servings:x
Cooking Time:x
Ingredients:
- 3 tsp. lemon juice
- 2 tbsp. coriander powder
- 3 tbsp. chopped capsicum
- 2 tbsp. peanut flour
- 2 cups cubed cottage cheese
- 3 onions chopped
- 5 green chilies-roughly chopped
- 1 ½ tbsp. ginger paste
- 1 ½ tsp. garlic paste
- 1 ½ tsp. salt
- 3 eggs

Directions:
1. Coat the cottage cheese cubes with the corn flour and mix the other ingredients in a bowl. Make the mixture into a smooth paste and coat the cheese cubes with the mixture. Beat the eggs in a bowl and add a little salt to them.
2. Dip the cubes in the egg mixture and coat them with sesame seeds and leave them in the refrigerator for an hour.
3. Pre heat the oven at 290 Fahrenheit for around 5 minutes. Place the kebabs in the basket and let them cook for another 25 minutes at the same temperature. Turn the kebabs over in between the cooking process to get a uniform cook. Serve the kebabs with mint sauce.

364.Lemony Wax Beans

Servings:4
Cooking Time: 12 Minutes
Ingredients:
- 2 pounds (907 g) wax beans

- 2 tablespoons extra-virgin olive oil
- Salt and freshly ground black pepper, to taste
- Juice of ½ lemon, for serving

Directions:
1. Line the air fryer basket with aluminum foil.
2. Toss the wax beans with the olive oil in a large bowl. Lightly season with salt and pepper.
3. Spread out the wax beans in the basket.
4. Put the air fryer basket on the baking pan and slide into Rack Position 2, select Roast, set temperature to 400ºF (205ºC), and set time to 12 minutes.
5. When done, the beans will be caramelized and tender. Remove from the oven to a plate and serve sprinkled with the lemon juice.

365.Vegetable Spicy Lemon Kebab

Servings:x
Cooking Time:x
Ingredients:
- 1 ½ tsp. salt
- 3 tsp. lemon juice
- 2 tsp. garam masala
- 4 tbsp. chopped coriander
- 3 tbsp. cream
- 3 tbsp. chopped capsicum
- 2 cups mixed vegetables
- 3 onions chopped
- 5 green chilies-roughly chopped
- 1 ½ tbsp. ginger paste
- 1 ½ tsp. garlic paste
- 3 eggs
- 2 ½ tbsp. white sesame seeds

Directions:
1. Grind the ingredients except for the egg and form a smooth paste. Coat the vegetables in the paste. Now, beat the eggs and add a little salt to it.
2. Dip the coated vegetables in the egg mixture and then transfer to the sesame seeds and coat the vegetables well. Place the vegetables on a stick.
3. Pre heat the oven at 160 degrees Fahrenheit for around 5 minutes. Place the sticks in the basket and let them cook for another 25 minutes at the same temperature. Turn the sticks over in between the cooking process to get a uniform cook.

366.Asian-inspired Broccoli

Servings:2
Cooking Time: 10 Minutes
Ingredients:
- 12 ounces (340 g) broccoli florets
- 2 tablespoons Asian hot chili oil

- 1 teaspoon ground Sichuan peppercorns (or black pepper)
- 2 garlic cloves, finely chopped
- 1 (2-inch) piece fresh ginger, peeled and finely chopped
- Kosher salt and freshly ground black pepper

Directions:
1. Toss the broccoli florets with the chili oil, Sichuan peppercorns, garlic, ginger, salt, and pepper in a mixing bowl until thoroughly coated.
2. Transfer the broccoli florets to the air fryer basket.
3. Put the air fryer basket on the baking pan and slide into Rack Position 2, select Air Fry, set temperature to 375ºF (190ºC), and set time to 10 minutes.
4. Stir the broccoli florets halfway through the cooking time.
5. When cooking is complete, the broccoli florets should be lightly browned and tender. Remove the broccoli from the oven and serve on a plate.

367.Parsley Hearty Carrots

Servings: 3
Cooking Time: 25 Minutes
Ingredients:
- 2 tsp olive oil
- 2 shallots, chopped
- 3 carrots, sliced
- Salt to taste
- ¼ cup yogurt
- 2 garlic cloves, minced
- 3 tbsp parsley, chopped

Directions:
1. In a baking dish, mix olive oil, carrots, salt, garlic, shallots, parsley, and yogurt.
2. Place the dish in your and cook for 15 minutes on Bake function at 370 F. Serve with garlic mayo.

368.Rosemary Squash With Cheese

Servings: 2
Cooking Time: 20 Minutes
Ingredients:
- 1 pound (454 g) butternut squash, cut into wedges
- 2 tablespoons olive oil
- 1 tablespoon dried rosemary
- Salt, to salt
- 1 cup crumbled goat cheese
- 1 tablespoon maple syrup

Directions:
1. Toss the squash wedges with the olive oil, rosemary, and salt in a large bowl until well coated.

2. Transfer the squash wedges to the air fryer basket, spreading them out in as even a layer as possible.
3. Put the air fryer basket on the baking pan and slide into Rack Position 2, select Air Fry, set temperature to 350ºF (180ºC), and set time to 20 minutes.
4. After 10 minutes, remove from the oven and flip the squash. Return the pan to the oven and continue cooking for 10 minutes.
5. When cooking is complete, the squash should be golden brown. Remove from the oven. Sprinkle the goat cheese on top and serve drizzled with the maple syrup.

369.Simple Ricotta & Spinach Balls

Servings: 4
Cooking Time: 20 Minutes
Ingredients:
- 14 oz store-bought crescent dough
- 1 cup steamed spinach
- 1 cup crumbled ricotta cheese
- ¼ tsp garlic powder
- 1 tsp chopped oregano
- ¼ tsp salt

Directions:
1. Preheat on Air Fry function to 350 F. Roll the dough onto a lightly floured flat surface. Combine the ricotta cheese, spinach, oregano, salt, and garlic powder together in a bowl. Cut the dough into 4 equal pieces.
2. Divide the spinach/feta mixture between the dough pieces. Make sure to place the filling in the center. Fold the dough and secure with a fork. Place onto a lined baking dish and then in your oven. Cook for 12 minutes until lightly browned. Serve.

370.Teriyaki Tofu

Servings:3
Cooking Time: 15 Minutes
Ingredients:
- Nonstick cooking spray
- 14 oz. firm or extra firm tofu, pressed & cut in 1-inch cubes
- ¼ cup cornstarch
- ½ tsp salt
- ½ tsp ginger
- ½ tsp white pepper
- 3 tbsp. olive oil
- 12 oz. bottle vegan teriyaki sauce

Directions:
1. Lightly spray baking pan with cooking spray.
2. In a shallow dish, combine cornstarch, salt, ginger, and pepper.
3. Heat oil in a large skillet over med-high heat.
4. Toss tofu cubes in cornstarch mixture then add to skillet. Cook 5 minutes, turning over halfway through, until tofu is nicely seared.

Transfer the tofu to the prepared baking pan.
5. Set oven to convection bake on 350°F for 15 minutes.
6. Pour all but ½ cup teriyaki sauce over tofu and stir to coat. After oven has preheated for 5 minutes, place the baking pan in position 2 and bake tofu 10 minutes.
7. Turn tofu over, spoon the sauce in the pan over it and bake another 10 minutes. Serve with reserved sauce for dipping.
- **Nutrition Info:** Calories 469, Total Fat 25g, Saturated Fat 4g, Total Carbs 33g, Net Carbs 30g, Protein 28g, Sugar 16g, Fiber 3g, Sodium 2424mg, Potassium 571mg, Phosphorus 428mg

371.Spicy Thai-style Vegetables

Servings:4
Cooking Time: 8 Minutes
Ingredients:
- 1 small head Napa cabbage, shredded, divided
- 1 medium carrot, cut into thin coins
- 8 ounces (227 g) snow peas
- 1 red or green bell pepper, sliced into thin strips
- 1 tablespoon vegetable oil
- 2 tablespoons soy sauce
- 1 tablespoon sesame oil
- 2 tablespoons brown sugar
- 2 tablespoons freshly squeezed lime juice
- 2 teaspoons red or green Thai curry paste
- 1 serrano chile, deseeded and minced
- 1 cup frozen mango slices, thawed
- ½ cup chopped roasted peanuts or cashews

Directions:
1. Put half the Napa cabbage in a large bowl, along with the carrot, snow peas, and bell pepper. Drizzle with the vegetable oil and toss to coat. Spread them evenly in the air fryer basket.
2. Put the air fryer basket on the baking pan and slide into Rack Position 2, select Roast, set temperature to 375ºF (190ºC), and set time to 8 minutes.
3. Meanwhile, whisk together the soy sauce, sesame oil, brown sugar, lime juice, and curry paste in a small bowl.
4. When done, the vegetables should be tender and crisp. Remove from the oven and put the vegetables back into the bowl. Add the chile, mango slices, and the remaining cabbage. Pour over the dressing and toss to coat. Top with the roasted nuts and serve.

372.Tortellini With Veggies And Parmesan

Servings:4
Cooking Time: 16 Minutes

Ingredients:

- 8 ounces (227 g) sugar snap peas, trimmed
- ½ pound (227 g) asparagus, trimmed and cut into 1-inch pieces
- 2 teaspoons kosher salt or 1 teaspoon fine salt, divided
- 1 tablespoon extra-virgin olive oil
- 1½ cups water
- 1 (20-ounce / 340-g) package frozen cheese tortellini
- 2 garlic cloves, minced
- 1 cup heavy (whipping) cream
- 1 cup cherry tomatoes, halved
- ½ cup grated Parmesan cheese
- ¼ cup chopped fresh parsley or basil
- Add the peas and asparagus to a large bowl. Add ½ teaspoon of kosher salt and the olive oil and toss until well coated. Place the veggies in the baking pan.

Directions:

1. Slide the baking pan into Rack Position 1, select Convection Bake, set the temperature to 450ºF (235ºC), and set the time for 4 minutes.
2. Meanwhile, dissolve 1 teaspoon of kosher salt in the water.
3. Once cooking is complete, remove the pan from the oven and place the tortellini in the pan. Pour the salted water over the tortellini. Put the pan back to the oven.
4. Slide the baking pan into Rack Position 1, select Convection Bake, set temperature to 450ºF (235ºC), and set time for 7 minutes.
5. Meantime, stir together the garlic, heavy cream, and remaining ½ teaspoon of kosher salt in a small bowl.
6. Once cooking is complete, remove the pan from the oven. Blot off any remaining water with a paper towel. Gently stir the ingredients. Drizzle the cream over and top with the tomatoes.
7. Slide the baking pan into Rack Position 2, select Roast, set the temperature to 375ºF (190ºC), and set the time for 5 minutes.
8. After 4 minutes, remove from the oven.
9. Add the Parmesan cheese and stir until the cheese is melted
10. Serve topped with the parsley.

373.Onion French Cuisine Galette

Servings:x
Cooking Time:x
Ingredients:

- 2 or 3 green chilies finely chopped
- 1 ½ tbsp. lemon juice
- Salt and pepper to taste
- 2 tbsp. garam masala
- 2 medium onions (Cut long)
- 1 ½ cup coarsely crushed peanuts

- 3 tsp. ginger finely chopped
- 1-2 tbsp. fresh coriander leaves

Directions:

1. Mix the ingredients in a clean bowl.
2. Mold this mixture into round and flat French Cuisine Galettes.
3. Wet the French Cuisine Galettes slightly with water. Coat each French Cuisine Galette with the crushed peanuts.
4. Pre heat the oven at 160 degrees Fahrenheit for 5 minutes. Place the French Cuisine Galettes in the fry basket and let them cook for another 25 minutes at the same temperature. Keep rolling them over to get a uniform cook. Serve either with mint sauce or ketchup.

374.Okra Flat Cakes

Servings:x
Cooking Time:x
Ingredients:

- 2 or 3 green chilies finely chopped
- 1 ½ tbsp. lemon juice
- Salt and pepper to taste
- 2 tbsp. garam masala
- 2 cups sliced okra
- 3 tsp. ginger finely chopped
- 1-2 tbsp. fresh coriander leaves

Directions:

1. Mix the ingredients in a clean bowl and add water to it. Make sure that the
2. paste is not too watery but is enough to apply on the okra.
3. Pre heat the oven at 160 degrees Fahrenheit for 5 minutes. Place the French Cuisine Galettes in the fry basket and let them cook for another 25 minutes at the same temperature. Keep rolling them over to get a uniform cook. Serve either with mint sauce or ketchup.

375.Tasty Polenta Crisps

Servings: 4
Cooking Time: 25 Minutes + Chilling Time
Ingredients:

- 2 cups milk
- 1 cup instant polenta
- Salt and black pepper to taste
- fresh thyme, chopped

Directions:

1. Fill a saucepan with milk and 2 cups of water and place over low heat. Bring to a simmer. Keep whisking as you pour in the polenta. Continue to whisk until polenta thickens and bubbles; season to taste. Add polenta to a lined with parchment paper baking tray and spread out.
2. Refrigerate for 45 minutes. Slice, set polenta into batons, and spray with olive oil.

Arrange polenta chips into the basket and fit in the baking tray; cook for 16 minutes at 380 F on Air Fry function, turning once halfway through. Make sure the fries are golden and crispy. Serve.

376.Stuffed Eggplant Baskets

Servings:x
Cooking Time:x
Ingredients:
- 1 tsp. cumin powder
- Salt and pepper to taste
- 3 tbsp. grated cheese
- 1 tsp. red chili flakes
- ½ tsp. oregano
- 6 eggplants
- ½ tsp. salt
- ½ tsp. pepper powder
- 1 medium onion finely chopped
- 1 green chili finely chopped
- 1 ½ tbsp. chopped coriander leaves
- 1 tsp. fenugreek
- 1 tsp. dried mango powder
- ½ tsp. basil
- ½ tsp. parsley

Directions:
1. Take all the ingredients under the heading "Filling" and mix them together in a bowl.
2. Remove the stem of the eggplant. Cut off the caps. Remove a little of the flesh as well. Sprinkle some salt and pepper on the inside of the capsicums.
3. Leave them aside for some time.
4. Now fill the eggplant with the filling prepared but leave a small space at the top. Sprinkle grated cheese and also add the seasoning.
5. Pre heat the oven at 140 degrees Fahrenheit for 5 minutes. Put the capsicums in the fry basket and close it. Let them cook at the same temperature for another 20 minutes. Turn them over in between to prevent over cooking.

377.Rosemary Butternut Squash Roast

Servings: 2
Cooking Time: 30 Minutes
Ingredients:
- 1 butternut squash
- 1 tbsp dried rosemary
- 2 tbsp maple syrup
- Salt to taste

Directions:
1. Place the squash on a cutting board and peel. Cut in half and remove the seeds and pulp. Slice into wedges and season with salt. Preheat on Air Fry function to 350 F. Spray the wedges with cooking spray and sprinkle with rosemary. Place the wedges in the

basket without overlapping and fit in the baking tray. Cook for 20 minutes, flipping once halfway through. Serve with maple syrup and goat cheese.

378.Herbed Broccoli With Cheese

Servings:4
Cooking Time: 18 Minutes
Ingredients:
- 1 large-sized head broccoli, stemmed and cut into small florets
- 2½ tablespoons canola oil
- 2 teaspoons dried basil
- 2 teaspoons dried rosemary
- Salt and ground black pepper, to taste
- $^1/_3$ cup grated yellow cheese

Directions:
1. Bring a pot of lightly salted water to a boil. Add the broccoli florets to the boiling water and let boil for about 3 minutes.
2. Drain the broccoli florets well and transfer to a large bowl. Add the canola oil, basil, rosemary, salt, and black pepper to the bowl and toss until the broccoli is fully coated. Place the broccoli in the air fryer basket.
3. Put the air fryer basket on the baking pan and slide into Rack Position 2, select Air Fry, set temperature to 390ºF (199ºC), and set time to 15 minutes.
4. Stir the broccoli halfway through the cooking time.
5. When cooking is complete, the broccoli should be crisp. Serve the broccoli warm with grated cheese sprinkled on top.

379.Cheese And Garlic French Fries

Servings:x
Cooking Time:x
Ingredients:
- 1 cup molten cheese
- 2 tsp. garlic powder
- 1 tbsp. lemon juice
- 2 medium sized potatoes peeled and cut into thick pieces lengthwise
- ingredients for the marinade:
- 1 tbsp. olive oil
- 1 tsp. mixed herbs
- ½ tsp. red chili flakes
- A pinch of salt to taste

Directions:
1. Boil the potatoes and blanch them. Cut the potato into Oregano Fingers. Mix the ingredients for the marinade and add the potato Oregano Fingers to it making sure that they are coated well.
2. Pre heat the oven for around 5 minutes at 300 Fahrenheit. Take out the basket of the

fryer and place the potato Oregano Fingers in them. Close the basket.

3. Now keep the fryer at 200 Fahrenheit for 20 or 25 minutes. In between the process, toss the fries twice or thrice so that they get cooked properly.

380.Gourd French Cuisine Galette

Servings:x
Cooking Time:x
Ingredients:
- 2 or 3 green chilies finely chopped
- 1 ½ tbsp. lemon juice
- Salt and pepper to taste
- 2 tbsp. garam masala
- 2 cups sliced gourd
- 1 ½ cup coarsely crushed peanuts
- 3 tsp. ginger finely chopped
- 1-2 tbsp. fresh coriander leaves

Directions:
1. Mix the ingredients in a clean bowl.
2. Mold this mixture into round and flat French Cuisine Galettes.
3. Wet the French Cuisine Galettes slightly with water. Coat each French Cuisine Galette with the crushed peanuts.
4. Pre heat the oven at 160 degrees Fahrenheit for 5 minutes. Place the French Cuisine Galettes in the fry basket and let them cook for another 25 minutes at the same temperature. Keep rolling them over to get a uniform cook. Serve either with mint sauce or ketchup

381.Coconut Vegan Fries

Servings: 2
Cooking Time: 20 Minutes
Ingredients:
- 2 potatoes, spiralized
- 1 tbsp tomato ketchup
- 2 tbsp olive oil
- Salt and black pepper to taste
- 2 tbsp coconut oil

Directions:
1. In a bowl, mix olive oil, coconut oil, salt, and pepper. Add in the potatoes and toss to coat. Place them in the basket and fit in the baking tray; cook for 15 minutes on Air Fry function at 360 F. Serve with ketchup and enjoy!

382.Cauliflower Spicy Lemon Kebab

Servings:x
Cooking Time:x
Ingredients:
- 3 tsp. lemon juice
- 2 tsp. garam masala
- 3 eggs
- 2 ½ tbsp. white sesame seeds
- 2 cups cauliflower florets
- 3 onions chopped
- 5 green chilies-roughly chopped
- 1 ½ tbsp. ginger paste
- 1 ½ tsp. garlic paste
- 1 ½ tsp. salt

Directions:
1. Grind the ingredients except for the egg and form a smooth paste. Coat the florets in the paste. Now, beat the eggs and add a little salt to it.
2. Dip the coated florets in the egg mixture and then transfer to the sesame seeds and coat the florets well. Place the vegetables on a stick.
3. Pre heat the oven at 160 degrees Fahrenheit for around 5 minutes. Place the sticks in the basket and let them cook for another 25 minutes at the same temperature. Turn the sticks over in between the cooking process to get a uniform cook.

383.Vegetable Skewer

Servings:x
Cooking Time:x
Ingredients:
- 3 tbsp. cream
- 3 eggs
- 2 cups mixed vegetables
- 3 onions chopped
- 5 green chilies
- 1 ½ tbsp. ginger paste
- 1 ½ tsp. garlic paste
- 1 ½ tsp. salt
- 2 ½ tbsp. white sesame seeds

Directions:
1. Grind the ingredients except for the egg and form a smooth paste. Coat the vegetables in the paste. Now, beat the eggs and add a little salt to it.
2. Dip the coated vegetables in the egg mixture and then transfer to the sesame seeds and coat the vegetables well. Place the vegetables on a stick.
3. Pre heat the oven at 160 degrees Fahrenheit for around 5 minutes. Place the sticks in the basket and let them cook for another 25 minutes at the same temperature. Turn the sticks over in between the cooking process to get a uniform cook.

384.Stuffed Portobello Mushrooms With Vegetables

Servings:4
Cooking Time: 8 Minutes
Ingredients:
- 4 portobello mushrooms, stem removed

- 1 tablespoon olive oil
- 1 tomato, diced
- ½ green bell pepper, diced
- ½ small red onion, diced
- ½ teaspoon garlic powder
- Salt and black pepper, to taste
- ½ cup grated Mozzarella cheese

Directions:
1. Using a spoon to scoop out the gills of the mushrooms and discard them. Brush the mushrooms with the olive oil.
2. In a mixing bowl, stir together the remaining ingredients except the Mozzarella cheese. Using a spoon to stuff each mushroom with the filling and scatter the Mozzarella cheese on top.
3. Arrange the mushrooms in the air fryer basket.
4. Put the air fryer basket on the baking pan and slide into Rack Position 2, select Roast, set temperature to 330ºF (166ºC) and set time to 8 minutes.
5. When cooking is complete, the cheese should be melted.
6. Serve warm.

385.Mushroom Club Sandwich

Servings:x
Cooking Time:x
Ingredients:
- ¼ tbsp. Worcestershire sauce
- ½ tsp. olive oil
- ½ flake garlic crushed
- ¼ cup chopped onion
- ¼ tbsp. red chili sauce
- ½ cup water
- 2 slices of white bread
- 1 tbsp. softened butter
- 1 cup minced mushroom
- 1 small capsicum

Directions:
1. Take the slices of bread and remove the edges. Now cut the slices horizontally.
2. Cook the ingredients for the sauce and wait till it thickens. Now, add the mushroom to the sauce and stir till it obtains the flavors. Roast the capsicum and peel the skin off. Cut the capsicum into slices. Apply the sauce on the slices.
3. Pre-heat the oven for 5 minutes at 300 Fahrenheit. Open the basket of the Fryer and place the prepared Classic Sandwiches in it such that no two Classic Sandwiches are touching each other. Now keep the fryer at 250 degrees for around 15 minutes. Turn the Classic Sandwiches in between the cooking process to cook both slices. Serve the Classic Sandwiches with tomato ketchup or mint sauce.

386.Traditional Jacket Potatoes

Servings: 4
Cooking Time: 30 Minutes
Ingredients:
- 4 potatoes, well washed
- 2 garlic cloves, minced
- Salt and black pepper to taste
- 1 tsp rosemary
- 1 tsp butter

Directions:
1. Preheat your Oven to 360 F on Air Fry function. Prick the potatoes with a fork. Place them into your Air fryer basket and fit in the baking tray; cook for 25 minutes. Cut the potatoes in half and top with butter and rosemary; season with salt and pepper. Serve immediately.

387.Tofu & Pea Cauli Rice

Servings:4
Cooking Time: 30 Minutes
Ingredients:
- Tofu:
- ½ block tofu
- ½ cup onions, chopped
- 2 tbsp soy sauce
- 1 tsp turmeric
- 1 cup carrots, chopped
- Cauliflower:
- 3 cups cauliflower rice
- 2 tbsp soy sauce
- ½ cup broccoli, chopped
- 2 garlic cloves, minced
- 1 ½ tsp toasted sesame oil
- 1 tbsp fresh ginger, minced
- ½ cup frozen peas
- 1 tbsp rice vinegar

Directions:
1. Preheat on AirFry function to 370 F. Crumble the tofu and combine it with all tofu ingredients. Place in a baking dish and cook for 10 minutes.
2. Meanwhile, place all cauliflower ingredients in a large bowl; mix to combine. Add the cauliflower mixture to the tofu and stir to combine. Press Start and cook for 12 minutes. Serve.

388.Crispy Potato Lentil Nuggets

Servings: 4
Cooking Time: 10 Minutes
Ingredients:
- Nonstick cooking spray
- 1 cup red lentils
- 1 tbsp. olive oil
- 1 cup onion, grated
- 1 cup carrot, grated
- 1 cup potato, grated

- ½ cup flour
- ½ tsp salt
- ½ tsp garlic powder
- ¾ tsp paprika
- ¼ tsp pepper

Directions:

1. Place baking pan in position 2. Lightly spray fryer basket with cooking spray.
2. Soak lentils in just enough water to cover them for 25 minutes.
3. Heat oil in a large skillet over medium heat. Add onion, carrot, and potato. Cook, stirring frequently until vegetables are tender, 12-15 minutes.
4. Drain the lentils and place them in a food processor. Add flour and spices and pulse to combine, leave some texture to the mixture.
5. Add cooked veggies to the food processor and pulse just until combined. Mixture will be sticky, so oil your hands. Form mixture into nugget shapes and add to the fryer basket in a single layer.
6. Place basket in the oven and set air fry on 350°F for 10 minutes. Turn nuggets over halfway through cooking time. Repeat with remaining mixture. Serve with your favorite dipping sauce.
- **Nutrition Info:** Calories 317, Total Fat 5g, Saturated Fat 1g, Total Carbs 54g, Net Carbs 46g, Protein 14g, Sugar 3g, Fiber 8g, Sodium 317mg, Potassium 625mg, Phosphorus 197mg

389.Roasted Bell Peppers With Garlic

Servings:4
Cooking Time: 22 Minutes
Ingredients:

- 1 green bell pepper, sliced into 1-inch strips
- 1 red bell pepper, sliced into 1-inch strips
- 1 orange bell pepper, sliced into 1-inch strips
- 1 yellow bell pepper, sliced into 1-inch strips
- 2 tablespoons olive oil, divided
- ½ teaspoon dried marjoram
- Pinch salt
- Freshly ground black pepper, to taste
- 1 head garlic

Directions:

1. Toss the bell peppers with 1 tablespoon of olive oil in a large bowl until well coated. Season with the marjoram, salt, and pepper. Toss again and set aside.
2. Cut off the top of a head of garlic. Place the garlic cloves on a large square of aluminum foil. Drizzle the top with the remaining 1 tablespoon of olive oil and wrap the garlic cloves in foil.
3. Transfer the garlic to the air fryer basket.
4. Put the air fryer basket on the baking pan and slide into Rack Position 2, select Roast, set temperature to 330ºF (166ºC) and set time to 15 minutes.
5. After 15 minutes, remove from the oven and add the bell peppers. Return to the oven and set time to 7 minutes.
6. When cooking is complete or until the garlic is soft and the bell peppers are tender.
7. Transfer the cooked bell peppers to a plate. Remove the garlic and unwrap the foil. Let the garlic rest for a few minutes. Once cooled, squeeze the roasted garlic cloves out of their skins and add them to the plate of bell peppers. Stir well and serve immediately.

390.Aloo Marinade Cutlet

Servings:x
Cooking Time:x
Ingredients:

- 4 tsp. fennel
- 2 tbsp. ginger-garlic paste
- 1 small onion
- 6-7 flakes garlic (optional)
- Salt to taste
- 4 medium potatoes (cut them into cubes)
- 1 big capsicum (Cut this capsicum into big cubes)
- 1 onion (Cut it into quarters. Now separate the layers carefully.)
- 5 tbsp. gram flour
- A pinch of salt to taste
- 2 cup fresh green coriander
- ½ cup mint leaves
- 3 tbsp. lemon juice

Directions:

1. Take a clean and dry container. Put into it the coriander, mint, fennel, and ginger, onion/garlic, salt and lemon juice. Mix them.
2. Pour the mixture into a grinder and blend until you get a thick paste. Now move on to the potato pieces. Slit these pieces almost till the end and leave them aside. Now stuff all the pieces with the paste that was obtained from the previous step. Now leave the stuffed potato aside. Take the sauce and add to it the gram flour and some salt. Mix them together properly. Rub this mixture all over the stuffed potato pieces.
3. Now leave the cottage cheese aside. Now, to the leftover sauce, add the capsicum and onions. Apply the sauce generously on each of the pieces of capsicum and onion. Now take satay sticks and arrange the potato pieces and vegetables on separate sticks. Pre heat the oven at 290 Fahrenheit for around 5 minutes.

4. Open the basket. Arrange the satay sticks properly. Close the basket. Keep the sticks with the cottage cheese at 180 degrees for around half an hour while the sticks with the vegetables are to be kept at the same temperature for only 7 minutes. Turn the sticks in between so that one side does not get burnt and also to provide a uniform cook.

391.Mixed Vegetable Patties

Servings:x
Cooking Time:x
Ingredients:
- 1 tbsp. fresh coriander leaves
- ¼ tsp. red chili powder
- ¼ tsp. cumin powder
- 2.55 Cottage cheese Momo's Recipe
- 1 ½ cup all-purpose flour
- ½ tsp. salt
- 1 cup grated mixed vegetables
- A pinch of salt to taste
- ¼ tsp. ginger finely chopped
- 1 green chili finely chopped
- 1 tsp. lemon juice
- 5 tbsp. water
- 2 cups crumbled cottage cheese
- 2 tbsp. oil
- 2 tsp. ginger-garlic paste
- 2 tsp. soya sauce
- 2 tsp. vinegar

Directions:
1. Squeeze the dough and cover it with plastic wrap and set aside. Next, cook the ingredients for the filling and try to ensure that the cottage cheese is covered well with the sauce.
2. Roll the dough and cut it into a square. Place the filling in the center. Now, wrap the dough to cover the filling and pinch the edges together.
3. Pre heat the oven at 200° F for 5 minutes. Place the gnocchi's in the fry basket and close it. Let them cook at the same temperature for another 20 minutes. Recommended sides are chili sauce or ketchup.
4. Mix the ingredients together and ensure that the flavors are right. You will now make round patties with the mixture and roll them out well.
5. Pre heat the oven at 250 Fahrenheit for 5 minutes. Open the basket of the Fryer and arrange the patties in the basket. Close it carefully. Keep the fryer at 150 degrees for around 10 or 12 minutes. In between the cooking process, turn the patties over to get a uniform cook. Serve hot with mint sauce.

392.Maple And Pecan Granola

Servings:4
Cooking Time: 20 Minutes
Ingredients:
- 1½ cups rolled oats
- ¼ cup maple syrup
- ¼ cup pecan pieces
- 1 teaspoon vanilla extract
- ½ teaspoon ground cinnamon

Directions:
1. Line a baking sheet with parchment paper.
2. Mix together the oats, maple syrup, pecan pieces, vanilla, and cinnamon in a large bowl and stir until the oats and pecan pieces are completely coated. Spread the mixture evenly in the baking pan.
3. Slide the baking pan into Rack Position 1, select Convection Bake, set temperature to 300ºF (150ºC), and set time to 20 minutes.
4. Stir once halfway through the cooking time.
5. When done, remove from the oven and cool for 30 minutes before serving. The granola may still be a bit soft right after removing, but it will gradually firm up as it cools.

393.Mozzarella Eggplant Patties

Servings: 1
Cooking Time: 10 Minutes
Ingredients:
- 1 hamburger bun
- 1 eggplant, sliced
- 1 mozzarella slice, chopped
- 1 red onion cut into 3 rings
- 1 lettuce leaf
- ½ tbsp tomato sauce
- 1 pickle, sliced

Directions:
1. Preheat on Bake function to 330 F. Place the eggplant slices in a greased baking tray and cook for 6 minutes. Take out the tray and top the eggplant with mozzarella cheese and cook for 30 more seconds. Spread tomato sauce on one half of the bun. Place the lettuce leaf on top of the sauce. Place the cheesy eggplant on top of the lettuce. Top with onion rings and pickles and then with the other bun half to serve.

394.Cauliflower Gnocchi's

Servings:x
Cooking Time:x
Ingredients:
- 2 tbsp. oil
- 2 tsp. ginger-garlic paste
- 2 tsp. soya sauce
- 2 tsp. vinegar
- 1 ½ cup all-purpose flour
- ½ tsp. salt
- 5 tbsp. water

- 2 cups grated cauliflower

Directions:
1. Squeeze the dough and cover it with plastic wrap and set aside. Next, cook the ingredients for the filling and try to ensure that the cauliflower is covered well with the sauce.
2. Roll the dough and place the filling in the center. Now, wrap the dough to cover the filling and pinch the edges together.
3. Pre heat the oven at 200° F for 5 minutes. Place the gnocchi's in the fry basket and close it. Let them cook at the same temperature for another 20
4. minutes. Recommended sides are chili sauce or ketchup.

395.Carrots & Shallots With Yogurt

Servings:4
Cooking Time: 25 Minutes
Ingredients:
- 2 tsp olive oil
- 2 shallots, chopped
- 3 carrots, sliced
- Salt to taste
- ¼ cup yogurt
- 2 garlic cloves, minced
- 3 tbsp parsley, chopped

Directions:
1. In a bowl, mix sliced carrots, salt, garlic, shallots, parsley, and yogurt. Sprinkle with oil. Place the veggies in the basket and press Start. Cook for 15 minutes on AirFry function at 370 F. Serve with basil and garlic mayo.

396.Roasted Vegetables With Rice

Servings:4
Cooking Time: 12 Minutes
Ingredients:
- 2 teaspoons melted butter
- 1 cup chopped mushrooms
- 1 cup cooked rice
- 1 cup peas
- 1 carrot, chopped
- 1 red onion, chopped
- 1 garlic clove, minced
- Salt and black pepper, to taste
- 2 hard-boiled eggs, grated
- 1 tablespoon soy sauce

Directions:
1. Coat the baking pan with melted butter.
2. Stir together the mushrooms, cooked rice, peas, carrot, onion, garlic, salt, and pepper in a large bowl until well mixed. Pour the mixture into the prepared baking pan.
3. Slide the baking pan into Rack Position 2, select Roast, set temperature to 380ºF (193ºC), and set time to 12 minutes.

4. When cooking is complete, remove from the oven. Divide the mixture among four plates. Serve warm with a sprinkle of grated eggs and a drizzle of soy sauce.

397.Cottage Cheese And Mushroom Mexican Burritos

Servings:x
Cooking Time:x
Ingredients:
- ½ cup mushrooms thinly sliced
- 1 cup cottage cheese cut in too long and slightly thick Oregano Fingers
- A pinch of salt to taste
- ½ tsp. red chili flakes
- 1 tsp. freshly ground peppercorns
- ½ cup pickled jalapenos
- 1-2 lettuce leaves shredded.
- ½ cup red kidney beans (soaked overnight)
- ½ small onion chopped
- 1 tbsp. olive oil
- 2 tbsp. tomato puree
- ¼ tsp. red chili powder
- 1 tsp. of salt to taste
- 4-5 flour tortillas
- 1 or 2 spring onions chopped finely. Also cut the greens.
- Take one tomato. Remove the seeds and chop it into small pieces.
- 1 green chili chopped.
- 1 cup of cheddar cheese grated.
- 1 cup boiled rice (not necessary).
- A few flour tortillas to put the filing in.

Directions:
1. Cook the beans along with the onion and garlic and mash them finely.
2. Now, make the sauce you will need for the burrito. Ensure that you create a slightly thick sauce.
3. For the filling, you will need to cook the ingredients well in a pan and ensure that the vegetables have browned on the outside.
4. To make the salad, toss the ingredients together. Place the tortilla and add a layer of sauce, followed by the beans and the filling at the center. Before you roll it, you will need to place the salad on top of the filling.
5. Pre-heat the oven for around 5 minutes at 200 Fahrenheit. Open the fry basket and keep the burritos inside. Close the basket properly. Let the Air
6. Fryer remain at 200 Fahrenheit for another 15 minutes or so. Halfway through, remove the basket and turn all the burritos over in order to get a uniform cook.

398.Amazing Macadamia Delight

Servings:6
Cooking Time: 20 Minutes

Ingredients:
- 3 cups macadamia nuts
- 3 tbsp liquid smoke
- Salt to taste
- 2 tbsp molasses

Directions:
1. Preheat on Bake function to 360 F. In a bowl, add salt, liquid, molasses, and cashews and toss to coat. Place the cashews ina baking tray and press Start. Cook for 10 minutes, shaking the basket every 5 minutes. Serve.

399.Cottage Cheese Homemade Fried Sticks

Servings:x
Cooking Time:x
Ingredients:
- One or two poppadums'
- 4 or 5 tbsp. corn flour
- 1 cup of water
- 2 cups cottage cheese
- 1 big lemon-juiced
- 1 tbsp. ginger-garlic paste
- For seasoning, use salt and red chili powder in small amounts
- ½ tsp. carom

Directions:

1. Take the cottage cheese. Cut it into long pieces. Now, make a mixture of lemon juice, red chili powder, salt, ginger garlic paste and carom to use as a marinade. Let the cottage cheese pieces marinate in the mixture for some time and then roll them in dry corn flour. Leave them aside for around 20 minutes.
2. Take the poppadum into a pan and roast them. Once they are cooked, crush them into very small pieces. Now take another container and pour around 100 ml of water into it. Dissolve 2 tbsp. of corn flour in this water. Dip the cottage cheese pieces in this solution of corn flour and roll them on to the pieces of crushed poppadum so that the poppadum sticks to the cottage cheese
3. . Pre heat the oven for 10 minutes at 290 Fahrenheit. Then open the basket of the fryer and place the cottage cheese pieces inside it. Close the basket properly. Let the fryer stay at 160 degrees for another 20 minutes. Halfway through, open the basket and toss the cottage cheese around a bit to allow for uniform cooking. Once they are done, you can serve it either with ketchup or mint sauce. Another recommended side is mint sauce.

SNACKS AND DESSERTS RECIPES

400.Cheesy Zucchini Tots

Servings:8
Cooking Time: 6 Minutes
Ingredients:
- 2 medium zucchini (about 12 ounces / 340 g), shredded
- 1 large egg, whisked
- ½ cup grated pecorino romano cheese
- ½ cup panko bread crumbs
- ¼ teaspoon black pepper
- 1 clove garlic, minced
- Cooking spray

Directions:
1. Using your hands, squeeze out as much liquid from the zucchini as possible. In a large bowl, mix the zucchini with the remaining ingredients except the oil until well incorporated.
2. Make the zucchini tots: Use a spoon or cookie scoop to place tablespoonfuls of the zucchini mixture onto a lightly floured cutting board and form into 1-inch logs.
3. Spritz the air fryer basket with cooking spray. Place the zucchini tots in the pan.
4. Put the air fryer basket on the baking pan and slide into Rack Position 2, select Air Fry, set temperature to 375ºF (190ºC), and set time to 6 minutes.
5. When cooking is complete, the tots should be golden brown. Remove from the oven to a serving plate and serve warm.

401.Cheese And Leeks Dip

Servings: 6
Cooking Time: 15 Minutes
Ingredients:
- 2 spring onions; minced
- 4 leeks; sliced
- ¼ cup coconut cream
- 3 tbsp. coconut milk
- 2 tbsp. butter; melted
- Salt and white pepper to the taste

Directions:
1. In a pan that fits your air fryer, mix all the ingredients and whisk them well.
2. Introduce the pan in the fryer and cook at 390°F for 12 minutes. Divide into bowls and serve
- **Nutrition Info:** Calories: 204; Fat: 12g; Fiber: 2g; Carbs: 4g; Protein: 14g

402.Vegetable Kebabs

Servings: 3
Cooking Time: 10 Minutes
Ingredients:
- 1/2 onion, cut into 1-inch pieces
- 2 bell peppers, cut into 1-inch pieces
- 1 zucchini, cut into 1-inch pieces
- 1 eggplant, cut into 1-inch pieces
- Pepper
- Salt

Directions:
1. Fit the oven with the rack in position 2.
2. Thread veggie onto the skewers and season with pepper and salt.
3. Place skewers in the air fryer basket then place an air fryer basket in the baking pan.
4. Place a baking pan on the oven rack. Set to air fry at 390 F for 10 minutes.
5. Serve and enjoy.
- **Nutrition Info:** Calories 81 Fat 0.6 g Carbohydrates 18.9 g Sugar 10.5 g Protein 3.3 g Cholesterol 0 mg

403.Chocolate Donuts

Servings: 8-10
Cooking Time: 20 Minutes
Ingredients:
- (8-ounce) can jumbo biscuits
- Cooking oil
- Chocolate sauce, such as Hershey's

Directions:
1. Preparing the Ingredients. Separate the biscuit dough into 8 biscuits and place them on a flat work surface. Use a small circle cookie cutter or a biscuit cutter to cut a hole in the center of each biscuit. You can also cut the holes using a knife.
2. Spray the Oven rack/basket with cooking oil. Place the Rack on the middle-shelf of the air fryer oven.
3. Air Frying. Place 4 donuts in the air fryer oven. Do not stack. Spray with cooking oil. Cook for 4 minutes.
4. Open the air fryer oven and flip the donuts. Cook for an additional 4 minutes.
5. Remove the cooked donuts from the air fryer, then repeat steps 3 and 4 for the remaining 4 donuts.
6. Drizzle chocolate sauce over the donuts and enjoy while warm.
- **Nutrition Info:** CALORIES: 181; FAT:98G; PROTEIN:3G; FIBER:1G

404.Cheesy Roasted Jalapeño Poppers

Servings:8
Cooking Time: 15 Minutes
Ingredients:
- 6 ounces (170 g) cream cheese, at room temperature
- 4 ounces (113 g) shredded Cheddar cheese
- 1 teaspoon chili powder
- 12 large jalapeño peppers, deseeded and sliced in half lengthwise
- 2 slices cooked bacon, chopped

- ¼ cup panko bread crumbs
- 1 tablespoon butter, melted

Directions:
1. In a medium bowl, whisk together the cream cheese, Cheddar cheese and chili powder. Spoon the cheese mixture into the jalapeño halves and arrange them in the baking pan.
2. In a small bowl, stir together the bacon, bread crumbs and butter. Sprinkle the mixture over the jalapeño halves.
3. Slide the baking pan into Rack Position 2, select Roast, set temperature to 375ºF (190ºC) and set time to 15 minutes.
4. When cooking is complete, remove from the oven. Let the poppers cool for 5 minutes before serving.

405.Cheese Garlic Dip

Servings: 12
Cooking Time: 20 Minutes
Ingredients:
- 4 garlic cloves, minced
- 5 oz Asiago cheese, shredded
- 1 cup sour cream
- 1 cup mozzarella cheese, shredded
- 8 oz cream cheese, softened

Directions:
1. Fit the oven with the rack in position
2. Add all ingredients into the mixing bowl and mix until well combined.
3. Pour mixture into the baking dish.
4. Set to bake at 350 F for 25 minutes. After 5 minutes place the baking dish in the preheated oven.
5. Serve and enjoy.
- **Nutrition Info:** Calories 157 Fat 14.4 g Carbohydrates 1.7 g Sugar 0.1 g Protein 5.7 g Cholesterol 41 mg

406.Dark Chocolate Lava Cakes

Servings: 4
Cooking Time: 20 Minutes
Ingredients:
- 3 ½ oz butter, melted
- 3 ½ tbsp sugar
- 1 ½ tbsp self-rising flour
- 3 ½ oz dark chocolate, melted
- 2 eggs

Directions:
1. Grease 4 ramekins with butter. Preheat on Bake function to 375 F. Beat the eggs and sugar until frothy. Stir in butter and chocolate; gently fold in the flour. Divide the mixture between the ramekins and bake for 10 minutes. Let cool for 2 minutes before turning the cakes upside down onto serving plates.

407.Olive Garlic Puffs

Servings:x
Cooking Time:x
Ingredients:
- ¾ cup flour
- teaspoon pepper
- 30 garlic-stuffed olives
- 5 tablespoons butter, softened
- 1 (3-ounce) package cream cheese, softened
- 1½ cups grated sharp Cheddar cheese
- 1 teaspoon Worcestershire sauce

Directions:
1. In medium bowl, combine butter, cream cheese, and Cheddar cheese. Cream well until blended. Add Worcestershire sauce and mix until blended. Add flour and pepper and mix to form dough.
2. Form dough around each olive, covering olive completely. Flash freeze in single layer on baking sheets, then package in zipper-lock bags. Label bag and freeze.
3. To reheat: Place frozen puffs on baking sheet. Bake at 400ºF for 10 to 12 minutes or until hot, puffed, and golden brown.

408.Chocolate Tarts

Servings:x
Cooking Time:x
Ingredients:
- 1 tbsp. sliced cashew
- For Truffle filling:
- 1 ½ melted chocolate
- 1 cup fresh cream
- 3 tbsp. butter
- 1 ½ cup plain flour
- ½ cup cocoa powder
- 3 tbsp. unsalted butter
- 2 tbsp. powdered sugar
- 2 cups cold water

Directions:
1. In a large bowl, mix the flour, cocoa powder, butter and sugar with your Oregano Fingers. The mixture should resemble breadcrumbs. Squeeze the dough using the cold milk and wrap it and leave it to cool for ten minutes. Roll the dough out into the pie and prick the sides of the pie.
2. Mix the ingredients for the filling in a bowl. Make sure that it is a little thick. Add the filling to the pie and cover it with the second round.
3. Preheat the fryer to 300 Fahrenheit for five minutes. You will need to place the tin in the basket and cover it. When the pastry has turned golden brown, you will need to remove the tin and let it cool. Cut into slices and serve with a dollop of cream.

409.Lemon Bars

Servings: 8
Cooking Time: 35 Minutes
Ingredients:
- ½ cup butter, melted
- 1 cup erythritol
- 1 and ¾ cups almond flour
- 3 eggs, whisked
- Zest of 1 lemon, grated
- Juice of 3 lemons

Directions:
1. In a bowl, mix 1 cup flour with half of the erythritol and the butter, stir well and press into a baking dish that fits the air fryer lined with parchment paper.
2. Put the dish in your air fryer and cook at 350 degrees F for 10 minutes.
3. Meanwhile, in a bowl, mix the rest of the flour with the remaining erythritol and the other Ingredients: and whisk well.
4. Spread this over the crust, put the dish in the air fryer once more and cook at 350 degrees F for 25 minutes.
5. Cool down, cut into bars and serve.
- **Nutrition Info:** Calories 210, fat 12, fiber 1, carbs 4, protein 8

410.Margherita Pizza

Servings: 4
Cooking Time: 18 Minutes
Ingredients:
- 1 whole-wheat pizza crust
- 1/2 cup mozzarella cheese, grated
- 1/2 cup can tomatoes
- 2 tbsp olive oil
- 3 Roma tomatoes, sliced
- 10 basil leaves

Directions:
1. Fit the oven with the rack in position
2. Roll out whole wheat pizza crust using a rolling pin. Make sure the crust is ½-inch thick.
3. Sprinkle olive oil on top of pizza crust.
4. Spread can tomatoes over pizza crust.
5. Arrange sliced tomatoes and basil on pizza crust. Sprinkle grated cheese on top.
6. Place pizza on top of the oven rack and set to bake at 425 F for 23 minutes.
7. Slice and serve.
- **Nutrition Info:** Calories 126 Fat 7.9 g Carbohydrates 11.3 g Sugar 4.2 g Protein 3.6 g Cholesterol 2 mg

411.Coconut Cookies With Pecans

Servings:10
Cooking Time: 25 Minutes
Ingredients:
- 1½ cups coconut flour
- 1½ cups extra-fine almond flour
- ½ teaspoon baking powder
- $1/3$ teaspoon baking soda
- 3 eggs plus an egg yolk, beaten
- ¾ cup coconut oil, at room temperature
- 1 cup unsalted pecan nuts, roughly chopped
- ¾ cup monk fruit
- ¼ teaspoon freshly grated nutmeg
- $1/3$ teaspoon ground cloves
- ½ teaspoon pure vanilla extract
- ½ teaspoon pure coconut extract
- ⅛ teaspoon fine sea salt

Directions:
1. Line the baking pan with parchment paper.
2. Mix the coconut flour, almond flour, baking powder, and baking soda in a large mixing bowl.
3. In another mixing bowl, stir together the eggs and coconut oil. Add the wet mixture to the dry mixture.
4. Mix in the remaining ingredients and stir until a soft dough forms.
5. Drop about 2 tablespoons of dough on the parchment paper for each cookie and flatten each biscuit until it's 1 inch thick.
6. Slide the baking pan into Rack Position 1, select Convection Bake, set temperature to 370ºF (188ºC), and set time to 25 minutes.
7. When cooking is complete, the cookies should be golden and firm to the touch.
8. Remove from the oven to a plate. Let the cookies cool to room temperature and serve.

412.Breaded Bananas With Chocolate Sauce

Servings:6
Cooking Time: 7 Minutes
Ingredients:
- ¼ cup cornstarch
- ¼ cup plain bread crumbs
- 1 large egg, beaten
- 3 bananas, halved crosswise
- Cooking spray
- Chocolate sauce, for serving

Directions:
1. Place the cornstarch, bread crumbs, and egg in three separate bowls.
2. Roll the bananas in the cornstarch, then in the beaten egg, and finally in the bread crumbs to coat well.
3. Spritz the air fryer basket with cooking spray.
4. Arrange the banana halves in the basket and mist them with cooking spray.
5. Put the air fryer basket on the baking pan and slide into Rack Position 2, select Air Fry, set temperature to 350ºF (180ºC), and set time to 7 minutes.
6. After about 5 minutes, flip the bananas and continue to air fry for another 2 minutes.

7. When cooking is complete, remove the bananas from the oven to a serving plate. Serve with the chocolate sauce drizzled over the top.

413.Mini Crab Cakes

Servings:x
Cooking Time:x
Ingredients:
- ½ cup dried bread crumbs
- ½ cup mayonnaise
- ¼ cup minced green onions
- 3 tablespoons olive oil
- 1-pound canned lump crabmeat
- 1 cup fresh cilantro leaves
- ½ cup chopped walnuts
- ½ cup grated Romano cheese
- 2 tablespoons olive oil

Directions:
1. Drain crabmeat well and pick over to remove any cartilage. Set aside in large bowl. In food processor or blender, combine cilantro, walnuts, cheese, and 2 tablespoons olive oil (6 tablespoons for triple batch). Process or blend until mixture forms a paste. Stir into crabmeat.
2. Add bread crumbs, mayonnaise, and green onions to crab mixture. Stir to combine. Form into 2- inch patties about ½-inch thick. Flash freeze on baking sheet. When frozen solid, pack crab cakes in rigid containers, with waxed paper between the layers. Label crab cakes and freeze. Reserve remaining olive oil in pantry.
3. To thaw and reheat: Thaw crab cakes in refrigerator overnight. Heat 3 tablespoons olive oil (9 for triple batch) in large, heavy skillet over medium heat. Fry crab cakes until golden and hot, turning once, about 3 to 5 minutes on each side.

414.Healthy Sesame Bars

Servings: 16
Cooking Time: 15 Minutes
Ingredients:
- 1 1/4 cups sesame seeds
- 1/4 cup applesauce
- 3/4 cup coconut butter
- 10 drops liquid stevia
- 1/2 tsp vanilla
- Pinch of salt

Directions:
1. Fit the oven with the rack in position
2. In a large bowl, add applesauce, coconut butter, vanilla, liquid stevia, and sea salt and stir until well combined.
3. Add sesame seeds and stir to coat.
4. Pour mixture into a greased baking dish.

5. Set to bake at 350 F for 20 minutes. After 5 minutes place the baking dish in the preheated oven.
6. Cut into pieces and serve.
- **Nutrition Info:** Calories 136 Fat 12.4 g Carbohydrates 5.7 g Sugar 1.2 g Protein 2.8 g Cholesterol 0 mg

415.Cheesy Brussels Sprouts

Servings: 4
Cooking Time: 12 Minutes
Ingredients:
- 1 lb Brussels sprouts, cut stems and halved
- 1/4 cup parmesan cheese, grated
- 1 tbsp olive oil
- 1/4 tsp paprika
- 1/4 tsp chili powder
- 1/2 tsp garlic powder
- Pepper
- Salt

Directions:
1. Fit the oven with the rack in position 2.
2. Toss Brussels sprouts with remaining ingredients except for cheese and place in air fryer basket then place air fryer basket in baking pan.
3. Place a baking pan on the oven rack. Set to air fry at 350 F for 12 minutes.
4. Top with parmesan cheese and serve.
- **Nutrition Info:** Calories 100 Fat 5.2 g Carbohydrates 11 g Sugar 2.6 g Protein 5.8 g Cholesterol 4 mg

416.Walnut Zucchini Bread

Servings: 8
Cooking Time: 20 Minutes
Ingredients:
- 1½ cups all-purpose flour
- ½ teaspoon baking soda
- ½ teaspoon baking powder
- ½ tablespoon ground cinnamon
- ½ teaspoon salt
- 2¼ cups white sugar
- ½ cup vegetable oil
- 1½ eggs
- 1½ teaspoons vanilla extract
- 1 cup zucchini, grated
- ½ cup walnuts, chopped

Directions:
1. In a bowl and mix together the flour, baking powder, baking soda, cinnamon, and salt.
2. In another large bowl, add the sugar, oil, eggs, and vanilla extract and whisk until well combined.
3. Add the flour mixture and mix until just combined.
4. Gently, fold in the zucchini and walnuts.
5. Place the mixture into a lightly greased loaf pan.

6. Press "Power Button" of Air Fry Oven and turn the dial to select the "Air Crisp" mode.
7. Press the Time button and again turn the dial to set the cooking time to 20 minutes.
8. Now push the Temp button and rotate the dial to set the temperature at 320 degrees F.
9. Press "Start/Pause" button to start.
10. When the unit beeps to show that it is preheated, open the lid.
11. Arrange the pan in "Air Fry Basket" and insert in the oven.
12. Place the pan onto a wire rack to cool for about 10 minutes.
13. Carefully, invert the bread onto wire rack to cool completely before slicing.
14. Cut the bread into desired-sized slices and serve.
- **Nutrition Info:** Calories 483 Total Fat 19.3 g Saturated Fat 3.2 g Cholesterol 31mg Sodium 241 mg Total Carbs 76 g Fiber 1.6 g Sugar 56.8 g Protein 5.5 g

417.Carrot, Raisin & Walnut Bread

Servings: 8
Cooking Time: 35 Minutes
Ingredients:
- 2 cups all-purpose flour
- 1½ teaspoons ground cinnamon
- 2 teaspoons baking soda
- ½ teaspoon salt
- 3 eggs
- ½ cup sunflower oil
- ½ cup applesauce
- ¼ cup honey
- ¼ cup plain yogurt
- 2 teaspoons vanilla essence
- 2½ cups carrots, peeled and shredded
- ½ cup raisins
- ½ cup walnuts

Directions:
1. Line the bottom of a greased baking pan with parchment paper.
2. In a medium bowl, sift together the flour, baking soda, cinnamon and salt.
3. In a large bowl, add the eggs, oil, applesauce, honey and yogurt and with a hand-held mixer, mix on medium speed until well combined.
4. Add the eggs, one at a time and whisk well.
5. Add the vanilla and mix well.
6. Add the flour mixture and mix until just combined.
7. Fold in the carrots, raisins and walnuts.
8. Place the mixture into a lightly greased baking pan.
9. With a piece of foil, cover the pan loosely.
10. Press "Power Button" of Air Fry Oven and turn the dial to select the "Air Crisp" mode.

11. Press the Time button and again turn the dial to set the cooking time to 30 minutes.
12. Now push the Temp button and rotate the dial to set the temperature at 347 degrees F.
13. Press "Start/Pause" button to start.
14. When the unit beeps to show that it is preheated, open the lid.
15. Arrange the pan in "Air Fry Basket" and insert in the oven.
16. After 25 minutes of cooking, remove the foil.
17. Place the pan onto a wire rack to cool for about 10 minutes.
18. Carefully, invert the bread onto wire rack to cool completely before slicing.
19. Cut the bread into desired-sized slices and serve.
- **Nutrition Info:** Calories 441 Total Fat 20.3 g Saturated Fat 2.2 g Cholesterol 62mg Sodium 592 mg Total Carbs 57.6 g Fiber 5.7 g Sugar 23.7 g Protein 9.2 g

418.Air Fryer Biscuit Donuts

Servings: 4
Cooking Time: 5 Minutes
Ingredients:
- Coconut oil
- 1 can of biscuit dough, premade
- 1/2 cup of white sugar
- 1/2 cup of powdered sugar
- 2 tablespoons of melted butter
- 2 teaspoons of cinnamon

Directions:
1. Set the Instant Vortex on Air fryer to 350 degrees F for 5 minutes. Cut the dough with the biscuit cutter. Brush the coconut oil on the cooking tray and place the biscuits on it. Insert the cooking tray in the Vortex when it displays "Add Food". Flip the sides when it displays "Turn Food". Remove from the oven when cooking time is complete. Drizzle the melted butter over the donuts and coat with either the cinnamon-sugar mixture or the powdered sugar. Serve warm.
- **Nutrition Info:** Calories: 301 Cal Total Fat: 32.2 g Saturated Fat: 0 g Cholesterol: 0 mg Sodium: 0 mg Total Carbs: 25 g Fiber: 0 g Sugar: 0 g Protein: 8.8 g

419.Chocolate Paradise Cake

Servings: 6
Cooking Time: 15 Minutes
Ingredients:
- 2 eggs, beaten
- 2/3 cup sour cream
- 1 cup almond flour
- 2/3 cup swerve
- 1/3 cup coconut oil, softened
- 1/4 cup cocoa powder
- 2 tablespoons chocolate chips, unsweetened

- 1 ½ teaspoons baking powder
- 1 teaspoon vanilla extract
- 1/2 teaspoon pure rum extract
- Chocolate Frosting:
- 1/2 cup butter, softened
- 1/4 cup cocoa powder
- 1 cup powdered swerve
- 2 tablespoons milk

Directions:
1. Mix all ingredients for the chocolate cake with a hand mixer on low speed. Scrape the batter into a cake pan.
2. Bake at 330 degrees F for 25 to 30 minutes. Transfer the cake to a wire rack
3. Meanwhile, whip the butter and cocoa until smooth. Stir in the powdered swerve. Slowly and gradually, pour in the milk until your frosting reaches desired consistency.
4. Whip until smooth and fluffy; then, frost the cooled cake. Place in your refrigerator for a couple of hours. Serve well chilled.
- **Nutrition Info:** 433 Calories; 44g Fat; 8g Carbs; 5g Protein; 9g Sugars; 9g Fiber

420. Vanilla-lemon Cupcakes With Lemon Glaze

Servings: 6
Cooking Time: 30 Minutes
Ingredients:
- 1 cup flour
- ½ cup sugar
- 1 small egg
- 1 tsp lemon zest
- ¾ tsp baking powder
- ¼ tsp baking soda
- ½ tsp salt
- 2 tbsp vegetable oil
- ½ cup milk
- ½ tsp vanilla extract
- Glaze:
- ½ cup powdered sugar
- 2 tsp lemon juice

Directions:
1. Preheat on Bake function to 350 F. In a bowl, combine all dry muffin ingredients. In another bowl, whisk together the wet ingredients. Gently combine the two mixtures.
2. Divide the batter between 6 greased muffin tins. Place the tins in the oven and cook for 13 to 16 minutes. Whisk the powdered sugar with the lemon juice. Spread the glaze over the muffins.

421. Homemade Doughnuts

Servings: 4
Cooking Time: 25 Minutes
Ingredients:
- 8 oz self-rising flour

- 1 tsp baking powder
- ½ cup milk
- 2 ½ tbsp butter
- 1 egg
- 2 oz brown sugar

Directions:
1. Preheat on Bake function to 350 F. Beat the butter with the sugar until smooth. Whisk in the egg and milk. In a bowl, combine flour with baking powder. Fold in the butter mixture.
2. Form donut shapes and cut off the center with cookie cutters. Arrange on a lined baking sheet and cook in for 15 minutes. Serve with whipped cream or icing.

422. Marshmallow Pastries

Servings: 4
Cooking Time: 5 Minutes
Ingredients:
- 4 phyllo pastry sheets, thawed
- 2 oz. butter, melted
- ¼ cup chunky peanut butter
- 4 teaspoons marshmallow fluff
- Pinch of salt

Directions:
1. Brush 1 sheet of phyllo with butter.
2. Place a second sheet of phyllo on top of first one and brush it with butter.
3. Repeat until all 4 sheets are used.
4. Cut the phyllo layers in 4 (3x12-inch) strips.
5. Place 1 tablespoon of peanut butter and 1 teaspoon of marshmallow fluff on the underside of a strip of phyllo.
6. Carefully, fold the tip of sheet over the filling to make a triangle.
7. Fold repeatedly in a zigzag manner until the filling is fully covered.
8. Press "Power Button" of Air Fry Oven and turn the dial to select the "Air Fry" mode.
9. Press the Time button and again turn the dial to set the cooking time to 5 minutes.
10. Now push the Temp button and rotate the dial to set the temperature at 360 degrees F.
11. Press "Start/Pause" button to start.
12. When the unit beeps to show that it is preheated, open the lid.
13. Arrange the pastries in greased "Air Fry Basket" and insert in the oven.
14. Sprinkle with a pinch of salt and serve warm.
- **Nutrition Info:** Calories 248 Total Fat 20.5 g Saturated Fat 9.2 g Cholesterol 30 mg Sodium 268 mg Total Carbs 12.7 g Fiber 1.3 g Sugar 2.6 g Protein 5.2 g

423. Chestnuts Spinach Dip

Servings: 8
Cooking Time: 40 Minutes

Ingredients:
- 8 oz cream cheese, softened
- 1 cup mayonnaise
- 1 cup parmesan cheese, grated
- 1 cup frozen spinach, thawed and squeeze out all liquid
- 1/4 tsp garlic powder
- 1/2 cup onion, minced
- 1/3 cup water chestnuts, drained and chopped
- 1/2 tsp pepper

Directions:
1. Fit the oven with the rack in position
2. Spray air fryer baking dish with cooking spray.
3. Add all ingredients into the bowl and mix until well combined.
4. Transfer bowl mixture into the baking dish.
5. Set to bake at 300 F for 45 minutes. After 5 minutes place the baking dish in the preheated oven.
6. Serve and enjoy.
- **Nutrition Info:** Calories 220 Fat 19.8 g Carbohydrates 9.1 g Sugar 2.3 g Protein 2.7 g Cholesterol 39 mg

424.Mixed Berries With Pecan Streusel Topping

Servings:3
Cooking Time: 17 Minutes
Ingredients:
- ½ cup mixed berries
- Cooking spray
- Topping:
- 1 egg, beaten
- 3 tablespoons almonds, slivered
- 3 tablespoons chopped pecans
- 2 tablespoons chopped walnuts
- 3 tablespoons granulated Swerve
- 2 tablespoons cold salted butter, cut into pieces
- ½ teaspoon ground cinnamon

Directions:
1. Lightly spray the baking pan with cooking spray.
2. Make the topping: In a medium bowl, stir together the beaten egg, nuts, Swerve, butter, and cinnamon until well blended.
3. Put the mixed berries in the bottom of the baking pan and spread the topping over the top.
4. Slide the baking pan into Rack Position 1, select Convection Bake, set temperature to 340ºF (171ºC), and set time to 17 minutes.
5. When cooking is complete, the fruit should be bubbly and topping should be golden brown.
6. Allow to cool for 5 to 10 minutes before serving.

425.Shrimp And Artichoke Puffs

Servings:x
Cooking Time:x
Ingredients:
- 1 (10-ounce) package frozen artichoke hearts, thawed
- 1 (3-ounce) package cream cheese, softened
- 1 cup shredded Coda cheese
- ½ cup mayonnaise
- 1 tablespoon lemon juice
- 1 teaspoon dried basil leaves
- 6 slices whole wheat bread
- 2 shallots, chopped
- 1 tablespoon olive oil
- ½ pound cooked shrimp

Directions:
1. Preheat oven to 300ºF. Using a 2-inch cookie cutter, cut rounds from bread slices. Place rounds on a baking sheet and bake at 300ºF for 7 to 9 minutes, or until crisp, turning once. Remove from oven and cool on wire racks.
2. In a heavy skillet, cook shallots in olive oil over medium heat until tender. Remove from heat. Chop shrimp and add to skillet along with thawed, drained, and chopped artichoke hearts. Add both cheeses, mayonnaise, lemon juice, and basil; stir well to blend.
3. Spoon 1 tablespoon shrimp mixture onto each bread round, covering the top and mounding the filling. Flash freeze on baking sheets. When frozen solid, pack in rigid containers, with waxed paper between layers. Label puffs and freeze.
4. To reheat: Place frozen puffs on a baking sheet and bake at 400ºF for 10 to 12 minutes or until topping is hot and bubbling.

426.Cinnamon Apple Wedges

Servings:4
Cooking Time: 12 Minutes
Ingredients:
- 2 medium apples, cored and sliced into ¼-inch wedges
- 1 teaspoon canola oil
- 2 teaspoons peeled and grated fresh ginger
- ½ teaspoon ground cinnamon
- ½ cup low-fat Greek vanilla yogurt, for serving

Directions:
1. In a large bowl, toss the apple wedges with the canola oil, ginger, and cinnamon until evenly coated. Put the apple wedges in the air fryer basket.
2. Put the air fryer basket on the baking pan and slide into Rack Position 2, select Air Fry, set temperature to 360ºF (182ºC), and set time to 12 minutes.

3. When cooking is complete, the apple wedges should be crisp-tender. Remove the apple wedges from the oven and serve drizzled with the yogurt.

427.Cheesy Sweet Pepper Poppers

Servings: 10
Cooking Time: 15 Minutes
Ingredients:
- 2 tbsp cilantro, chopped
- 8 oz cream cheese
- 8 oz gouda cheese, grated
- 1 lb mini sweet peppers, halved
- 2 garlic cloves, minced
- 1/4 cup onion, grated
- 1/2 cup feta cheese, crumbled

Directions:
1. Fit the oven with the rack in position
2. Add all ingredients except peppers into the bowl and mix well to combine.
3. Stuff each pepper halves with cheese mixture and place in baking pan.
4. Set to bake at 425 F for 20 minutes. After 5 minutes place the baking pan in the preheated oven.
5. Serve and enjoy.
- **Nutrition Info:** Calories 186 Fat 15.8 g Carbohydrates 2.8 g Sugar 1.6 g Protein 8.6 g Cholesterol 57 mg

428.Almond Blueberry Bars

Servings: 4
Cooking Time: 50 Minutes
Ingredients:
- 1/4 cup blueberries
- 3 tbsp coconut oil
- 2 tbsp coconut flour
- 1/2 cup almond flour
- 3 tbsp water
- 1 tbsp chia seeds
- 1 tsp vanilla
- 1 tsp fresh lemon juice
- 2 tbsp erythritol
- 1/4 cup almonds, sliced
- 1/4 cup coconut flakes

Directions:
1. Fit the oven with the rack in position
2. Line baking dish with parchment paper and set aside.
3. In a small bowl, mix together water and chia seeds. Set aside.
4. In a bowl, combine together all ingredients. Add chia mixture and stir well.
5. Pour mixture into the prepared baking dish and spread evenly.
6. Set to bake at 300 F for 55 minutes. After 5 minutes place the baking dish in the preheated oven.
7. Slice and serve.

- **Nutrition Info:** Calories 208 Fat 18.2 g Carbohydrates 9.1 g Sugar 2.3 g Protein 3.6 g Cholesterol 0 mg

429.Green Chiles Nachos

Servings:6
Cooking Time: 10 Minutes
Ingredients:
- 8 ounces (227 g) tortilla chips
- 3 cups shredded Monterey Jack cheese, divided
- 2 (7-ounce / 198-g) cans chopped green chiles, drained
- 1 (8-ounce / 227-g) can tomato sauce
- ¼ teaspoon dried oregano
- ¼ teaspoon granulated garlic
- ¼ teaspoon freshly ground black pepper
- Pinch cinnamon
- Pinch cayenne pepper

Directions:
1. Arrange the tortilla chips close together in a single layer in the baking pan. Sprinkle 1½ cups of the cheese over the chips. Arrange the green chiles over the cheese as evenly as possible. Top with the remaining 1½ cups of the cheese.
2. Slide the baking pan into Rack Position 2, select Roast, set temperature to 375ºF (190ºC) and set time to 10 minutes.
3. Meanwhile, stir together the remaining ingredients in a bowl.
4. When cooking is complete, the cheese will be melted and starting to crisp around the edges of the pan. Remove from the oven. Drizzle the sauce over the nachos and serve warm.

430.Vanilla Chocolate Chip Cookies

Servings: 30 Cookies
Cooking Time: 22 Minutes
Ingredients:
- $^1/_3$ cup (80g) organic brown sugar
- $^1/_3$ cup (80g) organic cane sugar
- 4 ounces (112g) cashew-based vegan butter
- ½ cup coconut cream
- 1 teaspoon vanilla extract
- 2 tablespoons ground flaxseed
- 1 teaspoon baking powder
- 1 teaspoon baking soda
- Pinch of salt
- 2¼ cups (220g) almond flour
- ½ cup (90g) dairy-free dark chocolate chips

Directions:
1. Line the baking pan with parchment paper.
2. Mix together the brown sugar, cane sugar, and butter in a medium bowl or the bowl of a stand mixer. Cream together with a mixer.

3. Fold in the coconut cream, vanilla, flaxseed, baking powder, baking soda, and salt. Stir well.
4. Add the almond flour, a little at a time, mixing after each addition until fully incorporated. Stir in the chocolate chips with a spatula.
5. Scoop the dough into the prepared baking pan.
6. Slide the baking pan into Rack Position 1, select Convection Bake, set temperature to 325°F (160°C), and set the time to 22 minutes.
7. Bake until the cookies are golden brown.
8. When cooking is complete, transfer the baking pan onto a wire rack to cool completely before serving.

431.Almond Pecan Cookies

Servings: 16
Cooking Time: 20 Minutes
Ingredients:
- 1/2 cup butter
- 1 tsp vanilla
- 2 tsp gelatin
- 2/3 cup Swerve
- 1 cup pecans
- 1/3 cup coconut flour
- 1 cup almond flour

Directions:
1. Fit the oven with the rack in position
2. Add butter, vanilla, gelatin, swerve, coconut flour, and almond flour into the food processor and process until crumbs form.
3. Add pecans and process until chopped.
4. Make cookies from prepared mixture and place onto a parchment-lined baking pan.
5. Set to bake at 350 F for 25 minutes. After 5 minutes place the baking pan in the preheated oven.
6. Serve and enjoy.
- **Nutrition Info:** Calories 101 Fat 10.2 g Carbohydrates 1.4 g Sugar 0.3 g Protein 1.8 g Cholesterol 15 mg

432.Spicy Snack Mix

Servings:x
Cooking Time:x
Ingredients:
- ½ cup butter, melted
- 3 tablespoons Worcestershire sauce
- 2 teaspoons dried Italian seasoning
- ½ teaspoon crushed red pepper flakes
- 2 cups salted mixed nuts
- 2 cups small pretzels
- 2 cups potato sticks
- teaspoon white pepper

Directions:

1. Preheat oven to 300ºF. Pour nuts, pretzels, and potato sticks onto two cookie sheets with sides. In small saucepan, combine melted butter with remaining ingredients. Drizzle over the nut mixture. Toss to coat. Bake at 300ºF for 20 to 25 minutes, or until mixture is glazed and fragrant, stirring once during baking.
2. Cool snack mix and pack into zipper-lock bags. Label bags and freeze.
3. To thaw and reheat: Thaw at room temperature for 1 to 3 hours. Spread on baking sheet and reheat in 300ºF oven for 5 to 8 minutes, until crisp.

433.Rustic Blackberry Galette

Servings:x
Cooking Time:x
Ingredients:
- Pinch of salt
- ¼ tsp cinnamon
- 1 tsp vanilla extract
- 1 package store-bought puff pastry, thawed
- 1 egg white, slightly beaten
- 2 lbs. fresh blackberries, rinsed and dried
- ¾ cup granulated sugar
- 2 Tbsp fresh lime juice
- 2 tsp chopped fresh basil
- 1 tsp chopped fresh mint

Directions:
1. Preheat oven to 375°F.
2. Roll out puff pastry and place in greased oven. Allow pastry to hang over the sides slightly.
3. Toss together blackberries, sugar, lime juice, basil, mint, salt, cinnamon and vanilla extract.
4. Spread fruit mixture inside pastry dough in oven.
5. Fold pastry over the berries to cover edges and about ½ way up. Brush egg white over pastry.
6. Place the pot in oven and bake about 40 minutes, until pastry browns.

434.Easy Blackberry Cobbler

Servings:6
Cooking Time: 20 To 25 Minutes
Ingredients:
- 3 cups fresh or frozen blackberries
- 1¾ cups sugar, divided
- 1 teaspoon vanilla extract
- 8 tablespoons (1 stick) butter, melted
- 1 cup self-rising flour
- Cooking spray

Directions:
1. Spritz the baking pan with cooking spray.

2. Mix the blackberries, 1 cup of sugar, and vanilla in a medium bowl and stir to combine.
3. Stir together the melted butter, remaining sugar, and flour in a separate medium bowl.
4. Spread the blackberry mixture evenly in the prepared pan and top with the butter mixture.
5. Slide the baking pan into Rack Position 1, select Convection Bake, set temperature to 350ºF (180ºC), and set time to 25 minutes.
6. After about 20 minutes, check if the cobbler has a golden crust and you can't see any batter bubbling while it cooks. If needed, bake for another 5 minutes.
7. Remove from the oven and place on a wire rack to cool to room temperature. Serve immediately.

435. Tasty Gingersnap Cookies

Servings: 8
Cooking Time: 10 Minutes
Ingredients:
- 1 egg
- 1/2 tsp ground cinnamon
- 1/2 tsp ground ginger
- 1 tsp baking powder
- 3/4 cup erythritol
- 1/2 tsp vanilla
- 1/8 tsp ground cloves
- 1/4 tsp ground nutmeg
- 2/4 cup butter, melted
- 1 1/2 cups almond flour
- Pinch of salt

Directions:
1. Fit the oven with the rack in position
2. In a mixing bowl, mix together all dry ingredients.
3. In another bowl, mix together all wet ingredients.
4. Add dry ingredients to the wet ingredients and mix until a dough-like mixture is formed.
5. Cover and place in the refrigerator for 30 minutes.
6. Make cookies from dough and place onto a parchment-lined baking pan.
7. Set to bake at 350 F for 15 minutes. After 5 minutes place the baking pan in the preheated oven.
8. Serve and enjoy.
- **Nutrition Info:** Calories 142 Fat 14.7 g Carbohydrates 1.8 g Sugar 0.3 g Protein 2 g Cholesterol 51 mg

436. Choco – Chip Muffins

Servings:x
Cooking Time:x
Ingredients:

- 3 tsp. vinegar
- ½ cup chocolate chips
- ½ tsp. vanilla essence
- Muffin cups or butter paper cups
- 2 cups All-purpose flour
- 1 ½ cup milk
- ½ tsp. baking powder
- ½ tsp. baking soda
- 2 tbsp. butter
- 1 cup sugar

Directions:
1. Mix the ingredients together and use your Oregano Fingers to get a crumbly mixture.
2. Add the baking soda and the vinegar to the milk and mix continuously. Add this milk to the mixture and create a batter, which you will need to transfer to the muffin cups.
3. Preheat the fryer to 300 Fahrenheit for five minutes. You will need to place the muffin cups in the basket and cover it. Cook the muffins for fifteen minutes and check whether or not the muffins are cooked using a toothpick.
4. Remove the cups and serve hot.

437. Gooey Chocolate Fudge Cake

Servings:x
Cooking Time:x
Ingredients:
- 3 Tbsp cocoa powder
- ½ cup water
- ¼ cup whole milk
- 1 egg
- 1 tsp vanilla extract
- 1 cup flour
- ½ tsp baking soda
- 1 cup sugar
- Pinch of salt
- ½ cup vegetable oil

Directions:
1. Preheat the oven to 350°F.
2. In a large bowl, whisk flour, baking soda, sugar and salt.
3. Combine oil, cocoa powder and water in another bowl.
4. Whisk in flour mixture and pour into oven.
5. Incorporate milk, egg and vanilla into the batter.
6. Bake for 25 minutes, or until edges are set and center is only slightly jiggly.

438. Rosemary Roasted Almonds

Servings: 12
Cooking Time: 20 Minutes
Ingredients:
- 2 1/2 cups almonds
- 1 tbsp fresh rosemary, chopped
- 1 tbsp olive oil
- 2 ½ tbsp maple syrup

- 1/4 tsp cayenne
- 1/4 tsp ground coriander
- 1/4 tsp cumin
- 1/4 tsp chili powder
- Pinch of salt

Directions:
1. Fit the oven with the rack in position
2. Spray a baking tray with cooking spray and set aside.
3. In a mixing bowl, whisk together oil, cayenne, coriander, cumin, chili powder, rosemary, maple syrup, and salt.
4. Add almond and stir to coat.
5. Spread almonds in baking pan.
6. Set to bake at 325 F for 20 minutes. After 5 minutes place the baking pan in the preheated oven.
7. Serve and enjoy.
- **Nutrition Info:** Calories 137 Fat 11.2 g Carbohydrates 7.3 g Sugar 3.3 g Protein 4.2 g Cholesterol 0 mg

439.Garlicky Roasted Mushrooms

Servings:4
Cooking Time: 27 Minutes
Ingredients:
- 16 garlic cloves, peeled
- 2 teaspoons olive oil, divided
- 16 button mushrooms
- ½ teaspoon dried marjoram
- ⅛ teaspoon freshly ground black pepper
- 1 tablespoon white wine

Directions:
1. Place the garlic cloves in the baking pan and drizzle with 1 teaspoon of the olive oil. Toss to coat well.
2. Slide the baking pan into Rack Position 2, select Roast, set temperature to 350ºF (180ºC) and set time to 12 minutes.
3. When cooking is complete, remove from the oven. Stir in the mushrooms, marjoram and pepper. Drizzle with the remaining 1 teaspoon of the olive oil and the white wine. Toss to coat well. Return the pan to the oven.
4. Select Roast, set temperature to 350ºF (180ºC) and set time to 15 minutes.
5. Once done, the mushrooms and garlic cloves will be softened. Remove from the oven.
6. Serve warm.

440.Arugula Artichoke Dip

Servings: 6
Cooking Time: 25 Minutes
Ingredients:
- 15 oz artichoke hearts, drained
- 1 cup cheddar cheese, shredded
- 1 tbsp onion, minced
- 1/2 cup mayonnaise
- 1 tsp Worcestershire sauce
- 3 cups arugula, chopped

Directions:
1. Fit the oven with the rack in position
2. Add all ingredients into the blender and blend until smooth.
3. Pour artichoke mixture into air fryer baking dish.
4. Set to bake at 400 F for 30 minutes. After 5 minutes place the baking dish in the preheated oven.
5. Serve and enjoy.
- **Nutrition Info:** Calories 190 Fat 13 g Carbohydrates 13.1 g Sugar 2.5 g Protein 7.5 g Cholesterol 25 mg

441.Stuffed Mushrooms With Sour Cream

Servings: 12
Cooking Time: 8 Minutes
Ingredients:
- ¼ orange bell pepper, diced
- ¾ cup Cheddar cheese, shredded
- 12 mushrooms caps, stems diced
- ½ onion, diced
- ½ small carrot, diced
- ¼ cup sour cream

Directions:
1. Preheat the Air fryer to 350 degree F and grease a baking tray.
2. Place mushroom stems, onion, orange bell pepper and carrot over medium heat in a skillet.
3. Cook for about 5 minutes until softened and stir in ½ cup Cheddar cheese and sour cream.
4. Stuff this mixture in the mushroom caps and arrange them on the baking tray.
5. Top with rest of the cheese and place the baking tray in the Air fryer basket.
6. Cook for about 8 minutes until cheese is melted and serve warm.
- **Nutrition Info:** Calories: 43, Fat: 3.1g, Carbohydrates: 1.7g, Sugar: 1g, Protein: 2.4g, Sodium: 55mg

442.Spiced Apple Chips

Servings:4
Cooking Time: 10 Minutes
Ingredients:
- 4 medium apples (any type will work), cored and thinly sliced
- ¼ teaspoon nutmeg
- ¼ teaspoon cinnamon
- Cooking spray

Directions:
1. Place the apple slices in a large bowl and sprinkle the spices on top. Toss to coat.

2. Put the apple slices in the air fryer basket in a single layer and spray them with cooking spray.
3. Put the air fryer basket on the baking pan and slide into Rack Position 2, select Air Fry, set temperature to 360ºF (182ºC), and set time to 10 minutes.
4. Stir the apple slices halfway through.
5. When cooking is complete, the apple chips should be crispy. Transfer the apple chips to a paper towel-lined plate and rest for 5 minutes before serving.

443.Cuban Sandwiches

Servings: 4 Sandwiches
Cooking Time: 8 Minutes
Ingredients:
- 8 slices ciabatta bread, about ¼-inch thick
- Cooking spray
- 1 tablespoon brown mustard
- Toppings:
- 6 to 8 ounces (170 to 227 g) thinly sliced leftover roast pork
- 4 ounces (113 g) thinly sliced deli turkey
- $^1/_3$ cup bread and butter pickle slices
- 2 to 3 ounces (57 to 85 g) Pepper Jack cheese slices

Directions:
1. On a clean work surface, spray one side of each slice of bread with cooking spray. Spread the other side of each slice of bread evenly with brown mustard.
2. Top 4 of the bread slices with the roast pork, turkey, pickle slices, cheese, and finish with remaining bread slices. Transfer to the air fryer basket.
3. Put the air fryer basket on the baking pan and slide into Rack Position 2, select Air Fry, set temperature to 390ºF (199ºC), and set time to 8 minutes.
4. When cooking is complete, remove from the oven. Cool for 5 minutes and serve warm.

444.Classic Pound Cake

Servings:8
Cooking Time: 30 Minutes
Ingredients:
- 1 stick butter, at room temperature
- 1 cup Swerve
- 4 eggs
- 1½ cups coconut flour
- ½ cup buttermilk
- ½ teaspoon baking soda
- ½ teaspoon baking powder
- ¼ teaspoon salt
- 1 teaspoon vanilla essence
- A pinch of ground star anise
- A pinch of freshly grated nutmeg
- Cooking spray

Directions:
1. Spray the baking pan with cooking spray.
2. With an electric mixer or hand mixer, beat the butter and Swerve until creamy. One at a time, mix in the eggs and whisk until fluffy. Add the remaining ingredients and stir to combine.
3. Transfer the batter to the prepared baking pan.
4. Slide the baking pan into Rack Position 1, select Convection Bake, set temperature to 320ºF (160ºC), and set time to 30 minutes.
5. When cooking is complete, the center of the cake should be springy.
6. Allow the cake to cool in the pan for 10 minutes before removing and serving.

445.Peach-blueberry Tart

Servings:6 To 8
Cooking Time: 30 Minutes
Ingredients:
- 4 peaches, pitted and sliced
- 1 cup fresh blueberries
- 2 tablespoons cornstarch
- 3 tablespoons sugar
- 1 tablespoon freshly squeezed lemon juice
- Cooking spray
- 1 sheet frozen puff pastry, thawed
- 1 tablespoon nonfat or low-fat milk
- Confectioners' sugar, for dusting

Directions:
1. Add the peaches, blueberries, cornstarch, sugar, and lemon juice to a large bowl and toss to coat.
2. Spritz a round baking pan with cooking spray.
3. Unfold the pastry and put in the prepared baking pan.
4. Lay the peach slices on the pan, slightly overlapping them. Scatter the blueberries over the peach.
5. Drape the pastry over the outside of the fruit and press pleats firmly together. Brush the milk over the pastry.
6. Slide the baking pan into Rack Position 1, select Convection Bake, set temperature to 400ºF (205ºC), and set time to 30 minutes.
7. Bake until the crust is golden brown and the fruit is bubbling.
8. When cooking is complete, remove from the oven and allow to cool for 10 minutes.
9. Serve the tart with the confectioners' sugar sprinkled on top.

446.Tapioca Pudding

Servings:x
Cooking Time:x
Ingredients:
- 3 tbsp. powdered sugar

- 3 tbsp. unsalted butter
- 2 cups tapioca pearls
- 2 cups milk
- 2 tbsp. custard powder

Directions:
1. Boil the milk and the sugar in a pan and add the custard powder followed by the tapioca pearls and stir till you get a thick mixture.
2. Preheat the fryer to 300 Fahrenheit for five minutes. Place the dish in the basket and reduce the temperature to 250 Fahrenheit. Cook for ten minutes and set aside to cool.

447.Effortless Apple Pie

Servings: 4
Cooking Time: 30 Minutes
Ingredients:
- 4 apples, diced
- 2 oz butter, melted
- 2 oz sugar
- 1 oz brown sugar
- 2 tsp cinnamon
- 1 egg, beaten
- 3 large puff pastry sheets
- ¼ tsp salt

Directions:
1. Whisk white sugar, brown sugar, cinnamon, salt, and butter together. Place the apples in a greased baking pan and coat them with the sugar mixture. Place the baking dish in your and cook for 10 minutes at 350 F on Bake function.
2. Meanwhile, roll out the pastry on a floured flat surface, and cut each sheet into 6 equal pieces. Divide the apple filling between the pieces. Brush the edges of the pastry squares with the egg.
3. Fold them and seal the edges with a fork. Place on a lined baking sheet and cook in the fryer at 350 F for 8 minutes. Flip over, increase the temperature to 390 F, and cook for 2 more minutes.

448.Corn And Black Bean Salsa

Servings:4
Cooking Time: 10 Minutes
Ingredients:
- ½ (15-ounce / 425-g) can corn, drained and rinsed
- ½ (15-ounce / 425-g) can black beans, drained and rinsed
- ¼ cup chunky salsa
- 2 ounces (57 g) reduced-fat cream cheese, softened
- ¼ cup shredded reduced-fat Cheddar cheese
- ½ teaspoon paprika
- ½ teaspoon ground cumin

- Salt and freshly ground black pepper, to taste

Directions:
1. Combine the corn, black beans, salsa, cream cheese, Cheddar cheese, paprika, and cumin in a medium bowl. Sprinkle with salt and pepper and stir until well blended.
2. Pour the mixture into the baking pan.
3. Slide the baking pan into Rack Position 2, select Air Fry, set temperature to 325ºF (163ºC), and set time to 10 minutes.
4. When cooking is complete, the mixture should be heated through. Rest for 5 minutes and serve warm.

449.Keto Mixed Berry Crumble Pots

Servings: 6
Cooking Time: 15 Minutes
Ingredients:
- 2 ounces unsweetened mixed berries
- 1/2 cup granulated swerve
- 2 tablespoons golden flaxseed meal
- 1/4 teaspoon ground star anise
- 1/2 teaspoon ground cinnamon
- 1 teaspoon xanthan gum
- 2/3 cup almond flour
- 1 cup powdered swerve
- 1/2 teaspoon baking powder
- 1/3 cup unsweetened coconut, finely shredded
- 1/2 stick butter, cut into small pieces

Directions:
1. Toss the mixed berries with the granulated swerve, golden flaxseed meal, star anise, cinnamon, and xanthan gum. Divide between six custard cups coated with cooking spray.
2. In a mixing dish, thoroughly combine the remaining ingredients. Sprinkle over the berry mixture.
3. Bake in the preheated Air Fryer at 330 degrees F for 35 minutes. Work in batches if needed.
- **Nutrition Info:** 155 Calories; 13g Fat; 1g Carbs; 1g Protein; 8g Sugars; 6g Fiber

450.Currant Cookies

Servings: 6
Cooking Time: 15 Minutes
Ingredients:
- ½ cup currants
- ½ cup swerve
- 2 cups almond flour
- ½ cup ghee; melted
- 1 tsp. vanilla extract
- 2 tsp. baking soda

Directions:
1. Take a bowl and mix all the ingredients and whisk well.

2. Spread this on a baking sheet lined with parchment paper, put the pan in the air fryer and cook at 350°F for 30 minutes
3. Cool down; cut into rectangles and serve.
- **Nutrition Info:** Calories: 172; Fat: 5g; Fiber: 2g; Carbs: 3g; Protein: 5g

451.Delicious Banana Pastry With Berries

Servings:2
Cooking Time: 15 Minutes
Ingredients:
- 3 bananas, sliced
- 3 tbsp honey
- 2 puff pastry sheets, cut into thin strips
- Fresh berries to serve

Directions:
1. Preheat on AirFry function to 340 F. Place the banana slices into the cooking basket. Cover with the pastry strips and top with honey. Press Start and cook for 10-12 minutes on Bake function. Serve with fresh berries.

452.Toasted Coco Flakes

Servings: 4
Cooking Time: 15 Minutes
Ingredients:
- 1 cup unsweetened coconut flakes
- ¼ cup granular erythritol.
- 2 tsp. coconut oil
- ⅛ tsp. salt

Directions:
1. Toss coconut flakes and oil in a large bowl until coated. Sprinkle with erythritol and salt. Place coconut flakes into the air fryer basket.
2. Adjust the temperature to 300 Degrees F and set the timer for 3 minutes.
3. Toss the flakes when 1 minute remains. Add an extra minute if you would like a more golden coconut flake. Store in an airtight container up to 3 days.
- **Nutrition Info:** Calories: 165; Protein: 1.3g; Fiber: 2.7g; Fat: 15.5g; Carbs: 20.3g

453.Yogurt Cake(1)

Servings: 12
Cooking Time: 15 Minutes
Ingredients:
- 6 eggs, whisked
- 8 oz. Greek yogurt
- 9 oz. coconut flour
- 4 tbsp. stevia
- 1 tsp. vanilla extract
- 1 tsp. baking powder

Directions:
1. Take a bowl and mix all the ingredients and whisk well.

2. Pour this into a cake pan that fits the air fryer lined with parchment paper.
3. Put the pan in the air fryer and cook at 330°F for 30 minutes
- **Nutrition Info:** Calories: 181; Fat: 13g; Fiber: 2g; Carbs: 4g; Protein: 5g

454.Spicy Crab Dip

Servings: 4
Cooking Time: 10 Minutes
Ingredients:
- 1 cup crabmeat
- 2 cups cheese, grated
- 1/4 cup mayonnaise
- 2 tbsp parsley, chopped
- 2 tbsp fresh lemon juice
- 2 tbsp hot sauce
- 1/2 cup green onion, sliced
- 1/4 tsp pepper
- 1/2 tsp salt

Directions:
1. Fit the oven with the rack in position
2. Add all ingredients into the mixing bowl and mix well.
3. Pour mixture into the greased baking dish.
4. Set to bake at 400 F for 15 minutes. After 5 minutes place the baking dish in the preheated oven.
5. Serve and enjoy.
- **Nutrition Info:** Calories 313 Fat 23.9 g Carbohydrates 8.8 g Sugar 3.1 g Protein 16.2 g Cholesterol 67 mg

455.Yogurt Pumpkin Bread

Servings: 4
Cooking Time: 15 Minutes
Ingredients:
- 2 large eggs
- 8 tablespoons pumpkin puree
- 6 tablespoons banana flour
- 4 tablespoons honey
- 4 tablespoons plain Greek yogurt
- 2 tablespoons vanilla essence
- Pinch of ground nutmeg 6 tablespoons oats

Directions:
1. In a bowl, add in all the ingredients except oats and with a hand mixer, mix until smooth.
2. Add the oats and with a fork, mix well.
3. Grease and flour a loaf pan.
4. Place the mixture into the prepared loaf pan.
5. Press "Power Button" of Air Fry Oven and turn the dial to select the "Air Crisp" mode.
6. Press the Time button and again turn the dial to set the cooking time to 15 minutes.
7. Now push the Temp button and rotate the dial to set the temperature at 360 degrees F.
8. Press "Start/Pause" button to start.

9. When the unit beeps to show that it is preheated, open the lid.
10. Arrange the pan in "Air Fry Basket" and insert in the oven.
11. Carefully, invert the bread onto wire rack to cool completely before slicing.
12. Cut the bread into desired-sized slices and serve.
- **Nutrition Info:** Calories 232 Total Fat 8.33 g Saturated Fat 1.5 g Cholesterol 94 mg Sodium 53 mg Total Carbs 29.3 g Fiber 2.8 g Sugar 20.5 g Protein 7.7 g

456.Orange Coconut Cake

Servings:6
Cooking Time: 17 Minutes
Ingredients:
- 1 stick butter, melted
- ¾ cup granulated Swerve
- 2 eggs, beaten
- ¾ cup coconut flour
- ¼ teaspoon salt
- $1/3$ teaspoon grated nutmeg
- $1/3$ cup coconut milk
- 1¼ cups almond flour
- ½ teaspoon baking powder
- 2 tablespoons unsweetened orange jam
- Cooking spray

Directions:
1. Coat the baking pan with cooking spray. Set aside.
2. In a large mixing bowl, whisk together the melted butter and granulated Swerve until fluffy.
3. Mix in the beaten eggs and whisk again until smooth. Stir in the coconut flour, salt, and nutmeg and gradually pour in the coconut milk. Add the remaining ingredients and stir until well incorporated.
4. Scrape the batter into the baking pan.
5. Slide the baking pan into Rack Position 1, select Convection Bake, set temperature to 355ºF (179ºC), and set time to 17 minutes.
6. When cooking is complete, the top of the cake should spring back when gently pressed with your fingers.
7. Remove from the oven to a wire rack to cool. Serve chilled.

OTHER FAVORITE RECIPES

457. Southwest Seasoning

Servings: About ¾ Cups
Cooking Time: 0 Minutes
Ingredients:
- 3 tablespoons ancho chile powder
- 3 tablespoons paprika
- 2 tablespoons dried oregano
- 2 tablespoons freshly ground black pepper
- 2 teaspoons cayenne
- 2 teaspoons cumin
- 1 tablespoon granulated onion
- 1 tablespoon granulated garlic

Directions:
1. Stir together all the ingredients in a small bowl.
2. Use immediately or place in an airtight container in the pantry.

458. Ritzy Chicken And Vegetable Casserole

Servings:4
Cooking Time: 15 Minutes
Ingredients:
- 4 boneless and skinless chicken breasts, cut into cubes
- 2 carrots, sliced
- 1 yellow bell pepper, cut into strips
- 1 red bell pepper, cut into strips
- 15 ounces (425 g) broccoli florets
- 1 cup snow peas
- 1 scallion, sliced
- Cooking spray
- Sauce:
- 1 teaspoon Sriracha
- 3 tablespoons soy sauce
- 2 tablespoons oyster sauce
- 1 tablespoon rice wine vinegar
- 1 teaspoon cornstarch
- 1 tablespoon grated ginger
- 2 garlic cloves, minced
- 1 teaspoon sesame oil
- 1 tablespoon brown sugar

Directions:
1. Spritz the baking pan with cooking spray.
2. Combine the chicken, carrot, and bell peppers in a large bowl. Stir to mix well.
3. Combine the ingredients for the sauce in a separate bowl. Stir to mix well.
4. Pour the chicken mixture into the baking pan, then pour the sauce over. Stir to coat well.
5. Slide the baking pan into Rack Position 1, select Convection Bake, set temperature to 370ºF (188ºC) and set time to 13 minutes.
6. Add the broccoli and snow peas to the pan halfway through.

7. When cooking is complete, the vegetables should be tender.
8. Remove from the oven and sprinkle with sliced scallion before serving.

459. Traditional Latkes

Servings: 4 Latkes
Cooking Time: 10 Minutes
Ingredients:
- 1 egg
- 2 tablespoons all-purpose flour
- 2 medium potatoes, peeled and shredded, rinsed and drained
- ¼ teaspoon granulated garlic
- ½ teaspoon salt
- Cooking spray

Directions:
1. Spritz the air fryer basket with cooking spray.
2. Whisk together the egg, flour, potatoes, garlic, and salt in a large bowl. Stir to mix well.
3. Divide the mixture into four parts, then flatten them into four circles. Arrange the circles onto the basket and spritz with cooking spray.
4. Put the air fryer basket on the baking pan and slide into Rack Position 2, select Air Fry, set temperature to 380ºF (193ºC) and set time to 10 minutes.
5. Flip the latkes halfway through.
6. When cooked, the latkes will be golden brown and crispy. Remove from the oven and serve immediately.

460. Southwest Corn And Bell Pepper Roast

Servings:4
Cooking Time: 10 Minutes
Ingredients:
- Corn:
- 1½ cups thawed frozen corn kernels
- 1 cup mixed diced bell peppers
- 1 jalapeño, diced
- 1 cup diced yellow onion
- ½ teaspoon ancho chile powder
- 1 tablespoon fresh lemon juice
- 1 teaspoon ground cumin
- ½ teaspoon kosher salt
- Cooking spray
- For Serving:
- ¼ cup feta cheese
- ¼ cup chopped fresh cilantro
- 1 tablespoon fresh lemon juice

Directions:
1. Spritz the air fryer basket with cooking spray.

2. Combine the ingredients for the corn in a large bowl. Stir to mix well.
3. Pour the mixture into the basket.
4. Put the air fryer basket on the baking pan and slide into Rack Position 2, select Air Fry, set temperature to 375ºF (190ºC) and set time to 10 minutes.
5. Stir the mixture halfway through the cooking time.
6. When done, the corn and bell peppers should be soft.
7. Transfer them onto a large plate, then spread with feta cheese and cilantro. Drizzle with lemon juice and serve.

461.Broccoli, Carrot, And Tomato Quiche

Servings:4
Cooking Time: 14 Minutes
Ingredients:
- 4 eggs
- 1 teaspoon dried thyme
- 1 cup whole milk
- 1 steamed carrots, diced
- 2 cups steamed broccoli florets
- 2 medium tomatoes, diced
- ¼ cup crumbled feta cheese
- 1 cup grated Cheddar cheese
- 1 teaspoon chopped parsley
- Salt and ground black pepper, to taste
- Cooking spray

Directions:
1. Spritz the baking pan with cooking spray.
2. Whisk together the eggs, thyme, salt, and ground black pepper in a bowl and fold in the milk while mixing.
3. Put the carrots, broccoli, and tomatoes in the prepared baking pan, then spread with feta cheese and ½ cup Cheddar cheese. Pour the egg mixture over, then scatter with remaining Cheddar on top.
4. Slide the baking pan into Rack Position 1, select Convection Bake, set temperature to 350ºF (180ºC) and set time to 14 minutes.
5. When cooking is complete, the egg should be set and the quiche should be puffed.
6. Remove the quiche from the oven and top with chopped parsley, then slice to serve.

462.Parsnip Fries With Garlic-yogurt Dip

Servings:4
Cooking Time: 10 Minutes
Ingredients:
- 3 medium parsnips, peeled, cut into sticks
- ¼ teaspoon kosher salt
- 1 teaspoon olive oil
- 1 garlic clove, unpeeled
- Cooking spray
- Dip:
- ¼ cup plain Greek yogurt

- ⅛ teaspoon garlic powder
- 1 tablespoon sour cream
- ¼ teaspoon kosher salt
- Freshly ground black pepper, to taste

Directions:
1. Spritz the air fryer basket with cooking spray.
2. Put the parsnip sticks in a large bowl, then sprinkle with salt and drizzle with olive oil.
3. Transfer the parsnip into the basket and add the garlic.
4. Put the air fryer basket on the baking pan and slide into Rack Position 2, select Air Fry, set temperature to 360ºF (182ºC) and set time to 10 minutes.
5. Stir the parsnip halfway through the cooking time.
6. Meanwhile, peel the garlic and crush it. Combine the crushed garlic with the ingredients for the dip. Stir to mix well.
7. When cooked, the parsnip sticks should be crisp. Remove the parsnip fries from the oven and serve with the dipping sauce.

463.Baked Cherry Tomatoes With Basil

Servings:2
Cooking Time: 5 Minutes
Ingredients:
- 2 cups cherry tomatoes
- 1 clove garlic, thinly sliced
- 1 teaspoon olive oil
- ⅛ teaspoon kosher salt
- 1 tablespoon freshly chopped basil, for topping
- Cooking spray

Directions:
1. Spritz the baking pan with cooking spray and set aside.
2. In a large bowl, toss together the cherry tomatoes, sliced garlic, olive oil, and kosher salt. Spread the mixture in an even layer in the prepared pan.
3. Slide the baking pan into Rack Position 1, select Convection Bake, set temperature to 360ºF (182ºC) and set time to 5 minutes.
4. When cooking is complete, the tomatoes should be the soft and wilted.
5. Transfer to a bowl and rest for 5 minutes. Top with the chopped basil and serve warm.

464.Kale Chips With Soy Sauce

Servings:2
Cooking Time: 5 Minutes
Ingredients:
- 4 medium kale leaves, about 1 ounce (28 g) each, stems removed, tear the leaves in thirds
- 2 teaspoons soy sauce
- 2 teaspoons olive oil

Directions:
1. Toss the kale leaves with soy sauce and olive oil in a large bowl to coat well. Place the leaves in the baking pan.
2. Put the air fryer basket on the baking pan and slide into Rack Position 2, select Air Fry, set temperature to 400ºF (205ºC) and set time to 5 minutes.
3. Flip the leaves with tongs gently halfway through.
4. When cooked, the kale leaves should be crispy. Remove from the oven and serve immediately.

465.Garlicky Olive Stromboli

Servings:8
Cooking Time: 25 Minutes
Ingredients:
- 4 large cloves garlic, unpeeled
- 3 tablespoons grated Parmesan cheese
- ½ cup packed fresh basil leaves
- ½ cup marinated, pitted green and black olives
- ¼ teaspoon crushed red pepper
- ½ pound (227 g) pizza dough, at room temperature
- 4 ounces (113 g) sliced provolone cheese (about 8 slices)
- Cooking spray

Directions:
1. Spritz the air fryer basket with cooking spray. Put the unpeeled garlic in the basket.
2. Put the air fryer basket on the baking pan and slide into Rack Position 2, select Air Fry, set temperature to 370ºF (188ºC) and set time to 10 minutes.
3. When cooked, the garlic will be softened completely. Remove from the oven and allow to cool until you can handle.
4. Peel the garlic and place into a food processor with 2 tablespoons of Parmesan, basil, olives, and crushed red pepper. Pulse to mix well. Set aside.
5. Arrange the pizza dough on a clean work surface, then roll it out with a rolling pin into a rectangle. Cut the rectangle in half.
6. Sprinkle half of the garlic mixture over each rectangle half, and leave ½-inch edges uncover. Top them with the provolone cheese.
7. Brush one long side of each rectangle half with water, then roll them up. Spritz the basket with cooking spray. Transfer the rolls to the basket. Spritz with cooking spray and scatter with remaining Parmesan.
8. Select Air Fry and set time to 15 minutes.
9. Flip the rolls halfway through the cooking time. When done, the rolls should be golden brown.
10. Remove the rolls from the oven and allow to cool for a few minutes before serving.

466.Roasted Carrot Chips

Servings: 3 Cups
Cooking Time: 15 Minutes
Ingredients:
- 3 large carrots, peeled and sliced into long and thick chips diagonally
- 1 tablespoon granulated garlic
- 1 teaspoon salt
- ¼ teaspoon ground black pepper
- 1 tablespoon olive oil
- 1 tablespoon finely chopped fresh parsley

Directions:
1. Toss the carrots with garlic, salt, ground black pepper, and olive oil in a large bowl to coat well. Place the carrots in the air fryer basket.
2. Put the air fryer basket on the baking pan and slide into Rack Position 2, select Roast, set temperature to 360ºF (182ºC) and set time to 15 minutes.
3. Stir the carrots halfway through the cooking time.
4. When cooking is complete, the carrot chips should be soft. Remove from the oven. Serve the carrot chips with parsley on top.

467.Classic Marinara Sauce

Servings: About 3 Cups
Cooking Time: 30 Minutes
Ingredients:
- ¼ cup extra-virgin olive oil
- 3 garlic cloves, minced
- 1 small onion, chopped (about ½ cup)
- 2 tablespoons minced or puréed sun-dried tomatoes (optional)
- 1 (28-ounce / 794-g) can crushed tomatoes
- ½ teaspoon dried basil
- ½ teaspoon dried oregano
- ¼ teaspoon red pepper flakes

Directions:
1. 1 teaspoon kosher salt or ½ teaspoon fine salt, plus more as needed
2. Heat the oil in a medium saucepan over medium heat.
3. Add the garlic and onion and sauté for 2 to 3 minutes, or until the onion is softened. Add the sun-dried tomatoes (if desired) and cook for 1 minute until fragrant. Stir in the crushed tomatoes, scraping any brown bits from the bottom of the pot. Fold in the basil, oregano, red pepper flakes, and salt. Stir well.
4. Bring to a simmer. Cook covered for about 30 minutes, stirring occasionally.
5. Turn off the heat and allow the sauce to cool for about 10 minutes.

6. Taste and adjust the seasoning, adding more salt if needed.
7. Use immediately.

468.Chorizo, Corn, And Potato Frittata

Servings:4
Cooking Time: 12 Minutes
Ingredients:
- 2 tablespoons olive oil
- 1 chorizo, sliced
- 4 eggs
- ½ cup corn
- 1 large potato, boiled and cubed
- 1 tablespoon chopped parsley
- ½ cup feta cheese, crumbled
- Salt and ground black pepper, to taste

Directions:
1. Heat the olive oil in a nonstick skillet over medium heat until shimmering.
2. Add the chorizo and cook for 4 minutes or until golden brown.
3. Whisk the eggs in a bowl, then sprinkle with salt and ground black pepper.
4. Mix the remaining ingredients in the egg mixture, then pour the chorizo and its fat into the baking pan. Pour in the egg mixture.
5. Slide the baking pan into Rack Position 1, select Convection Bake, set temperature to 330ºF (166ºC) and set time to 8 minutes.
6. Stir the mixture halfway through.
7. When cooking is complete, the eggs should be set.
8. Serve immediately.

469.Chocolate And Coconut Macaroons

Servings: 24 Macaroons
Cooking Time: 8 Minutes
Ingredients:
- 3 large egg whites, at room temperature
- ¼ teaspoon salt
- ¾ cup granulated white sugar
- 4½ tablespoons unsweetened cocoa powder
- 2¼ cups unsweetened shredded coconut

Directions:
1. Line the air fryer basket with parchment paper.
2. Whisk the egg whites with salt in a large bowl with a hand mixer on high speed until stiff peaks form.
3. Whisk in the sugar with the hand mixer on high speed until the mixture is thick. Mix in the cocoa powder and coconut.
4. Scoop 2 tablespoons of the mixture and shape the mixture in a ball. Repeat with remaining mixture to make 24 balls in total.
5. Arrange the balls in a single layer in the basket and leave a little space between each two balls.

6. Put the air fryer basket on the baking pan and slide into Rack Position 2, select Air Fry, set temperature to 375ºF (190ºC) and set time to 8 minutes.
7. When cooking is complete, the balls should be golden brown.
8. Serve immediately.

470.Crunchy Green Tomatoes Slices

Servings: 12 Slices
Cooking Time: 8 Minutes
Ingredients:
- ½ cup all-purpose flour
- 1 egg
- ½ cup buttermilk
- 1 cup cornmeal
- 1 cup panko
- 2 green tomatoes, cut into ¼-inch-thick slices, patted dry
- ½ teaspoon salt
- ½ teaspoon ground black pepper
- Cooking spray

Directions:
1. Spritz a baking sheet with cooking spray.
2. Pour the flour in a bowl. Whisk the egg and buttermilk in a second bowl. Combine the cornmeal and panko in a third bowl.
3. Dredge the tomato slices in the bowl of flour first, then into the egg mixture, and then dunk the slices into the cornmeal mixture. Shake the excess off.
4. Transfer the well-coated tomato slices in the baking sheet and sprinkle with salt and ground black pepper. Spritz the tomato slices with cooking spray.
5. Put the air fryer basket on the baking pan and slide into Rack Position 2, select Air Fry, set temperature to 400ºF (205ºC) and set time to 8 minutes.
6. Flip the slices halfway through the cooking time.
7. When cooking is complete, the tomato slices should be crispy and lightly browned. Remove the baking sheet from the oven.
8. Serve immediately.

471.Easy Corn And Bell Pepper Casserole

Servings:4
Cooking Time: 20 Minutes
Ingredients:
- 1 cup corn kernels
- ¼ cup bell pepper, finely chopped
- ½ cup low-fat milk
- 1 large egg, beaten
- ½ cup yellow cornmeal
- ½ cup all-purpose flour
- ½ teaspoon baking powder
- 2 tablespoons melted unsalted butter
- 1 tablespoon granulated sugar

- Pinch of cayenne pepper
- ¼ teaspoon kosher salt
- Cooking spray

Directions:
1. Spritz the baking pan with cooking spray.
2. Combine all the ingredients in a large bowl. Stir to mix well. Pour the mixture into the baking pan.
3. Slide the baking pan into Rack Position 1, select Convection Bake, set temperature to 330ºF (166ºC) and set time to 20 minutes.
4. When cooking is complete, the casserole should be lightly browned and set.
5. Remove from the oven and serve immediately.

472.Dehydrated Honey-rosemary Roasted Almonds

Servings:x
Cooking Time:x
Ingredients:
- 1 heaping tablespoon demerara sugar
- 1 teaspoon finely chopped fresh rosemary
- 1 teaspoon kosher salt
- 8 ounces (225g) raw almonds
- 2 tablespoons kosher salt
- Honey-Rosemary glaze
- ¼ cup (80g) honey

Directions:
1. Place almonds and salt in a bowl. Add cold tap water to cover the almonds by 1-inch
2. (2cm). Let soak at room temperature for 12 hours to activate.
3. Rinse almonds under cold running water, then drain. Spread in a single layer on the dehydrate basket.
4. Dehydrate almonds for 24 hours or till tender and somewhat crispy but additionally spongy in the middle. Almonds may be eaten plain or roasted each the next recipe.
5. Put honey in a small saucepan and heat over Low heat. Put triggered nuts
6. At a medium bowl and then pour over warm honey. Stir To coat nuts equally. Add rosemary, sugar
7. And salt and stir to blend.
8. Spread Almonds in one layer on the skillet.
9. Insert cable rack into rack place 6. Select BAKE/350°F (175°C)/CONVECTION/10 moments and empower Rotate Remind.
10. Stirring almonds when Rotate Remind signs.
11. Let cool completely before storing in an airtight container.

473.Taco Beef And Chile Casserole

Servings:4
Cooking Time: 15 Minutes
Ingredients:
- 1 pound (454 g) 85% lean ground beef
- 1 tablespoon taco seasoning
- 1 (7-ounce / 198-g) can diced mild green chiles
- ½ cup milk
- 2 large eggs
- 1 cup shredded Mexican cheese blend
- 2 tablespoons all-purpose flour
- ½ teaspoon kosher salt
- Cooking spray

Directions:
1. Spritz the baking pan with cooking spray.
2. Toss the ground beef with taco seasoning in a large bowl to mix well. Pour the seasoned ground beef in the prepared baking pan.
3. Combing the remaining ingredients in a medium bowl. Whisk to mix well, then pour the mixture over the ground beef.
4. Slide the baking pan into Rack Position 1, select Convection Bake, set temperature to 350ºF (180ºC) and set time to 15 minutes.
5. When cooking is complete, a toothpick inserted in the center should come out clean.
6. Remove the casserole from the oven and allow to cool for 5 minutes, then slice to serve.

474.Corn On The Cob With Mayonnaise

Servings:4
Cooking Time: 10 Minutes
Ingredients:
- 2 tablespoons mayonnaise
- 2 teaspoons minced garlic
- ½ teaspoon sea salt
- 1 cup panko bread crumbs
- 4 (4-inch length) ears corn on the cob, husk and silk removed
- Cooking spray

Directions:
1. Spritz the air fryer basket with cooking spray.
2. Combine the mayonnaise, garlic, and salt in a bowl. Stir to mix well. Pour the panko on a plate.
3. Brush the corn on the cob with mayonnaise mixture, then roll the cob in the bread crumbs and press to coat well.
4. Transfer the corn on the cob in the basket and spritz with cooking spray.
5. Put the air fryer basket on the baking pan and slide into Rack Position 2, select Air Fry, set temperature to 400ºF (205ºC) and set time to 10 minutes.
6. Flip the corn on the cob at least three times during the cooking.
7. When cooked, the corn kernels on the cob should be almost browned. Remove from the oven and serve immediately.

475.Citrus Avocado Wedge Fries

Servings: 12 Fries
Cooking Time: 8 Minutes
Ingredients:
- 1 cup all-purpose flour
- 3 tablespoons lime juice
- ¾ cup orange juice
- 1¼ cups plain dried bread crumbs
- 1 cup yellow cornmeal
- 1½ tablespoons chile powder
- 2 large Hass avocados, peeled, pitted, and cut into wedges
- Coarse sea salt, to taste
- Cooking spray

Directions:
1. Spritz the air fryer basket with cooking spray.
2. Pour the flour in a bowl. Mix the lime juice with orange juice in a second bowl. Combine the bread crumbs, cornmeal, and chile powder in a third bowl.
3. Dip the avocado wedges in the bowl of flour to coat well, then dredge the wedges into the bowl of juice mixture, and then dunk the wedges in the bread crumbs mixture. Shake the excess off.
4. Arrange the coated avocado wedges in a single layer in the basket. Spritz with cooking spray.
5. Put the air fryer basket on the baking pan and slide into Rack Position 2, select Air Fry, set temperature to 400ºF (205ºC) and set time to 8 minutes.
6. Stir the avocado wedges and sprinkle with salt halfway through the cooking time.
7. When cooking is complete, the avocado wedges should be tender and crispy.
8. Serve immediately.

476.Shrimp With Sriracha And Worcestershire Sauce

Servings:4
Cooking Time: 10 Minutes
Ingredients:
- 1 tablespoon Sriracha sauce
- 1 teaspoon Worcestershire sauce
- 2 tablespoons sweet chili sauce
- ¾ cup mayonnaise
- 1 egg, beaten
- 1 cup panko bread crumbs
- 1 pound (454 g) raw shrimp, shelled and deveined, rinsed and drained
- Lime wedges, for serving
- Cooking spray

Directions:
1. Spritz the air fryer basket with cooking spray.
2. Combine the Sriracha sauce, Worcestershire sauce, chili sauce, and mayo in a bowl. Stir to mix well. Reserve $^1/_3$ cup of the mixture as the dipping sauce.
3. Combine the remaining sauce mixture with the beaten egg. Stir to mix well. Put the panko in a separate bowl.
4. Dredge the shrimp in the sauce mixture first, then into the panko. Roll the shrimp to coat well. Shake the excess off.
5. Place the shrimp in the basket, then spritz with cooking spray.
6. Put the air fryer basket on the baking pan and slide into Rack Position 2, select Air Fry, set temperature to 360ºF (182ºC) and set time to 10 minutes.
7. Flip the shrimp halfway through the cooking time.
8. When cooking is complete, the shrimp should be opaque.
9. Remove the shrimp from the oven and serve with reserve sauce mixture and squeeze the lime wedges over.

477.Air Fried Bacon Pinwheels

Servings: 8 Pinwheels
Cooking Time: 10 Minutes
Ingredients:
- 1 sheet puff pastry
- 2 tablespoons maple syrup
- ¼ cup brown sugar
- 8 slices bacon
- Ground black pepper, to taste
- Cooking spray

Directions:
1. Spritz the air fryer basket with cooking spray.
2. Roll the puff pastry into a 10-inch square with a rolling pin on a clean work surface, then cut the pastry into 8 strips.
3. Brush the strips with maple syrup and sprinkle with sugar, leaving a 1-inch far end uncovered.
4. Arrange each slice of bacon on each strip, leaving a ⅛-inch length of bacon hang over the end close to you. Sprinkle with black pepper.
5. From the end close to you, roll the strips into pinwheels, then dab the uncovered end with water and seal the rolls.
6. Arrange the pinwheels in the basket and spritz with cooking spray.
7. Put the air fryer basket on the baking pan and slide into Rack Position 2, select Air Fry, set temperature to 360ºF (182ºC) and set time to 10 minutes.
8. Flip the pinwheels halfway through.
9. When cooking is complete, the pinwheels should be golden brown. Remove from the oven and serve immediately.

478. Shawarma Spice Mix

Servings: About 1 Tablespoon
Cooking Time: 0 Minutes
Ingredients:

- 1 teaspoon smoked paprika
- 1 teaspoon cumin
- ¼ teaspoon turmeric
- ¼ teaspoon kosher salt or ⅛ teaspoon fine salt
- ¼ teaspoon cinnamon
- ¼ teaspoon allspice
- ¼ teaspoon red pepper flakes
- ¼ teaspoon freshly ground black pepper

Directions:
1. Stir together all the ingredients in a small bowl.
2. Use immediately or place in an airtight container in the pantry.

479. Herbed Cheddar Frittata

Servings: 4
Cooking Time: 20 Minutes
Ingredients:

- ½ cup shredded Cheddar cheese
- ½ cup half-and-half
- 4 large eggs
- 2 tablespoons chopped scallion greens
- 2 tablespoons chopped fresh parsley
- ½ teaspoon kosher salt
- ½ teaspoon ground black pepper
- Cooking spray

Directions:
1. Spritz the baking pan with cooking spray.
2. Whisk together all the ingredients in a large bowl, then pour the mixture into the prepared baking pan.
3. Slide the baking pan into Rack Position 1, select Convection Bake, set temperature to 300ºF (150ºC) and set time to 20 minutes.
4. Stir the mixture halfway through.
5. When cooking is complete, the eggs should be set.
6. Serve immediately.

480. Sweet Air Fried Pecans

Servings: 4 Cups
Cooking Time: 10 Minutes
Ingredients:

- 2 egg whites
- 1 tablespoon cumin
- 2 teaspoons smoked paprika
- ½ cup brown sugar
- 2 teaspoons kosher salt
- 1 pound (454 g) pecan halves
- Cooking spray

Directions:
1. Spritz the air fryer basket with cooking spray.

2. Combine the egg whites, cumin, paprika, sugar, and salt in a large bowl. Stir to mix well. Add the pecans to the bowl and toss to coat well.
3. Transfer the pecans to the basket.
4. Put the air fryer basket on the baking pan and slide into Rack Position 2, select Air Fry, set temperature to 300ºF (150ºC) and set time to 10 minutes.
5. Stir the pecans at least two times during the cooking.
6. When cooking is complete, the pecans should be lightly caramelized. Remove from the oven and serve immediately.

481. Jewish Blintzes

Servings: 8 Blintzes
Cooking Time: 10 Minutes
Ingredients:

- 2 (7½-ounce / 213-g) packages farmer cheese, mashed
- ¼ cup cream cheese
- ¼ teaspoon vanilla extract
- ¼ cup granulated white sugar
- 8 egg roll wrappers
- 4 tablespoons butter, melted

Directions:
1. Combine the farmer cheese, cream cheese, vanilla extract, and sugar in a bowl. Stir to mix well.
2. Unfold the egg roll wrappers on a clean work surface, spread ¼ cup of the filling at the edge of each wrapper and leave a ½-inch edge uncovering.
3. Wet the edges of the wrappers with water and fold the uncovered edge over the filling. Fold the left and right sides in the center, then tuck the edge under the filling and fold to wrap the filling.
4. Brush the wrappers with melted butter, then arrange the wrappers in a single layer in the air fryer basket, seam side down. Leave a little space between each two wrappers.
5. Put the air fryer basket on the baking pan and slide into Rack Position 2, select Air Fry, set temperature to 375ºF (190ºC) and set time to 10 minutes.
6. When cooking is complete, the wrappers will be golden brown.
7. Serve immediately.

482. Cheesy Green Bean Casserole

Servings: 4
Cooking Time: 6 Minutes
Ingredients:

- 1 tablespoon melted butter
- 1 cup green beans
- 6 ounces (170 g) Cheddar cheese, shredded

- 7 ounces (198 g) Parmesan cheese, shredded
- ¼ cup heavy cream
- Sea salt, to taste

Directions:
1. Grease the baking pan with the melted butter.
2. Add the green beans, Cheddar, salt, and black pepper to the prepared baking pan. Stir to mix well, then spread the Parmesan and cream on top.
3. Slide the baking pan into Rack Position 1, select Convection Bake, set temperature to 400ºF (205ºC) and set time to 6 minutes.
4. When cooking is complete, the beans should be tender and the cheese should be melted.
5. Serve immediately.

483.Oven Grits

Servings: About 4 Cups
Cooking Time: 1 Hour 5 Minutes
Ingredients:
- 1 cup grits or polenta (not instant or quick cook)
- 2 cups chicken or vegetable stock
- 2 cups milk
- 2 tablespoons unsalted butter, cut into 4 pieces
- 1 teaspoon kosher salt or ½ teaspoon fine salt

Directions:
1. Add the grits to the baking pan. Stir in the stock, milk, butter, and salt.
2. Select Bake, set the temperature to 325ºF (163ºC), and set the time for 1 hour and 5 minutes. Select Start to begin preheating.
3. Once the unit has preheated, place the pan in the oven.
4. After 15 minutes, remove the pan from the oven and stir the polenta. Return the pan to the oven and continue cooking.
5. After 30 minutes, remove the pan again and stir the polenta again. Return the pan to the oven and continue cooking for 15 to 20 minutes, or until the polenta is soft and creamy and the liquid is absorbed.
6. When done, remove the pan from the oven.
7. Serve immediately.

484.Butternut Squash With Hazelnuts

Servings: 3 Cups
Cooking Time: 23 Minutes
Ingredients:
- 2 tablespoons whole hazelnuts
- 3 cups butternut squash, peeled, deseeded and cubed
- ¼ teaspoon kosher salt
- ¼ teaspoon freshly ground black pepper
- 2 teaspoons olive oil

- Cooking spray

Directions:
1. Spritz the air fryer basket with cooking spray. Spread the hazelnuts in the pan.
2. Put the air fryer basket on the baking pan and slide into Rack Position 2, select Air Fry, set temperature to 300ºF (150ºC) and set time to 3 minutes.
3. When done, the hazelnuts should be soft. Remove from the oven. Chopped the hazelnuts roughly and transfer to a small bowl. Set aside.
4. Put the butternut squash in a large bowl, then sprinkle with salt and pepper and drizzle with olive oil. Toss to coat well. Transfer the squash to the lightly greased basket.
5. Put the air fryer basket on the baking pan and slide into Rack Position 2, select Air Fry, set temperature to 360ºF (182ºC) and set time to 20 minutes.
6. Flip the squash halfway through the cooking time.
7. When cooking is complete, the squash will be soft. Transfer the squash to a plate and sprinkle with the chopped hazelnuts before serving.

485.Dehydrated Crackers With Oats

Servings:x
Cooking Time:x
Ingredients:
- 3 tablespoons (20g) psyllium husk powder
- 2 teaspoons fine sea salt
- 1 teaspoon freshly ground black pepper
- 2 teaspoons ground turmeric, divided
- 3 tablespoons melted coconut oil
- 1 cup (125g) sunflower seeds
- ½ cup (75g) flaxseeds
- ¾ cup (50g) pumpkin seeds
- ¼ cup (35g) sesame seeds
- 2 tablespoons (30g) chia seeds
- 1½ cups (150g) rolled oats
- 1½ cups (360ml) water
- 1 large parsnip (10 ounces/300g), finely Grated

Directions:
1. In a large bowl Blend All of the seeds, Oats, psyllium husk, pepper, salt and 1 teaspoon ground turmeric.
2. Whisk coconut water and oil together in a measuring Cup. Add to the dry ingredients and blend well until all is totally saturated and dough becomes very thick.
3. Mix grated parsnip using 1 tsp turmeric and stir to blend.
4. Shape the first half to a disc and place it with a rolling pin, firmly roll dough to a thin sheet that the size of this dehydrate basket.

5. Put dough and parchment paper at the dehydrate basket.
6. Repeat steps 4 with remaining dough.
7. Hours and allow Rotate Remind. Place dehydrate baskets in rack positions 5 and 3. Press START.
8. Dehydrate crackers until tender. When prompted By Rotate Remind, rotate the baskets leading to back and change rack amounts.
9. Eliminate baskets out of oven and let rest for 10 minutes. Split crackers into shards.
10. Container for up to two months.

486.Smoked Trout And Crème Fraiche Frittata

Servings:4
Cooking Time: 17 Minutes
Ingredients:
- 2 tablespoons olive oil
- 1 onion, sliced
- 1 egg, beaten
- ½ tablespoon horseradish sauce
- 6 tablespoons crème fraiche
- 1 cup diced smoked trout
- 2 tablespoons chopped fresh dill
- Cooking spray

Directions:
1. Spritz the baking pan with cooking spray.
2. Heat the olive oil in a nonstick skillet over medium heat until shimmering.
3. Add the onion and sauté for 3 minutes or until translucent.
4. Combine the egg, horseradish sauce, and crème fraiche in a large bowl. Stir to mix well, then mix in the sautéed onion, smoked trout, and dill.
5. Pour the mixture in the prepared baking pan.
6. Slide the baking pan into Rack Position 1, select Convection Bake, set temperature to 350ºF (180ºC) and set time to 14 minutes.
7. Stir the mixture halfway through.
8. When cooking is complete, the egg should be set and the edges should be lightly browned.
9. Serve immediately.

487.Milky Pecan Tart

Servings:8
Cooking Time: 26 Minutes
Ingredients:
- Tart Crust:
- ¼ cup firmly packed brown sugar
- $^1/_3$ cup butter, softened
- 1 cup all-purpose flour
- ¼ teaspoon kosher salt
- Filling:
- ¼ cup whole milk

- 4 tablespoons butter, diced
- ½ cup packed brown sugar
- ¼ cup pure maple syrup
- 1½ cups finely chopped pecans
- ¼ teaspoon pure vanilla extract
- ¼ teaspoon sea salt

Directions:
1. Line the baking pan with aluminum foil, then spritz the pan with cooking spray.
2. Stir the brown sugar and butter in a bowl with a hand mixer until puffed, then add the flour and salt and stir until crumbled.
3. Pour the mixture in the prepared baking pan and tilt the pan to coat the bottom evenly.
4. Slide the baking pan into Rack Position 1, select Convection Bake, set temperature to 350ºF (180ºC) and set time to 13 minutes.
5. When done, the crust will be golden brown.
6. Meanwhile, pour the milk, butter, sugar, and maple syrup in a saucepan. Stir to mix well. Bring to a simmer, then cook for 1 more minute. Stir constantly.
7. Turn off the heat and mix the pecans and vanilla into the filling mixture.
8. Pour the filling mixture over the golden crust and spread with a spatula to coat the crust evenly.
9. Select Bake and set time to 12 minutes. When cooked, the filling mixture should be set and frothy.
10. Remove the baking pan from the oven and sprinkle with salt. Allow to sit for 10 minutes or until cooled.
11. Transfer the pan to the refrigerator to chill for at least 2 hours, then remove the aluminum foil and slice to serve.

488.Chicken Divan

Servings:4
Cooking Time: 24 Minutes
Ingredients:
- 4 chicken breasts
- Salt and ground black pepper, to taste
- 1 head broccoli, cut into florets
- ½ cup cream of mushroom soup
- 1 cup shredded Cheddar cheese
- ½ cup croutons
- Cooking spray

Directions:
1. Spritz the air fryer basket with cooking spray.
2. Put the chicken breasts in the basket and sprinkle with salt and ground black pepper.
3. Put the air fryer basket on the baking pan and slide into Rack Position 2, select Air Fry, set temperature to 390ºF (199ºC) and set time to 14 minutes.

4. Flip the breasts halfway through the cooking time.
5. When cooking is complete, the breasts should be well browned and tender.
6. Remove the breasts from the oven and allow to cool for a few minutes on a plate, then cut the breasts into bite-size pieces.
7. Combine the chicken, broccoli, mushroom soup, and Cheddar cheese in a large bowl. Stir to mix well.
8. Spritz the baking pan with cooking spray. Pour the chicken mixture into the pan. Spread the croutons over the mixture.
9. Slide the baking pan into Rack Position 1, select Convection Bake, set time to 10 minutes.
10. When cooking is complete, the croutons should be lightly browned and the mixture should be set.
11. Remove from the oven and serve immediately.

489.Kale Salad Sushi Rolls With Sriracha Mayonnaise

Servings:12
Cooking Time: 10 Minutes
Ingredients:
- Kale Salad:
- 1½ cups chopped kale
- 1 tablespoon sesame seeds
- ¾ teaspoon soy sauce
- ¾ teaspoon toasted sesame oil
- ½ teaspoon rice vinegar
- ¼ teaspoon ginger
- ⅛ teaspoon garlic powder
- Sushi Rolls:
- 3 sheets sushi nori
- 1 batch cauliflower rice
- ½ avocado, sliced
- Sriracha Mayonnaise:
- ¼ cup Sriracha sauce
- ¼ cup vegan mayonnaise
- Coating:
- ½ cup panko bread crumbs

Directions:
1. In a medium bowl, toss all the ingredients for the salad together until well coated and set aside.
2. Place a sheet of nori on a clean work surface and spread the cauliflower rice in an even layer on the nori. Scoop 2 to 3 tablespoon of kale salad on the rice and spread over. Place 1 or 2 avocado slices on top. Roll up the sushi, pressing gently to get a nice, tight roll. Repeat to make the remaining 2 rolls.
3. In a bowl, stir together the Sriracha sauce and mayonnaise until smooth. Add bread crumbs to a separate bowl.

4. Dredge the sushi rolls in Sriracha Mayonnaise, then roll in bread crumbs till well coated.
5. Place the coated sushi rolls in the air fryer basket.
6. Put the air fryer basket on the baking pan and slide into Rack Position 2, select Air Fry, set temperature to 390ºF (199ºC) and set time to 10 minutes.
7. Flip the sushi rolls halfway through the cooking time.
8. When cooking is complete, the sushi rolls will be golden brown and crispy. .
9. Transfer to a platter and rest for 5 minutes before slicing each roll into 8 pieces. Serve warm.

490.Air Fried Crispy Brussels Sprouts

Servings:4
Cooking Time: 20 Minutes
Ingredients:
- ¼ teaspoon salt
- ⅛ teaspoon ground black pepper
- 1 tablespoon extra-virgin olive oil
- 1 pound (454 g) Brussels sprouts, trimmed and halved
- Lemon wedges, for garnish

Directions:
1. Combine the salt, black pepper, and olive oil in a large bowl. Stir to mix well.
2. Add the Brussels sprouts to the bowl of mixture and toss to coat well. Arrange the Brussels sprouts in the air fryer basket.
3. Put the air fryer basket on the baking pan and slide into Rack Position 2, select Air Fry, set temperature to 350ºF (180ºC) and set time to 20 minutes.
4. Stir the Brussels sprouts two times during cooking.
5. When cooked, the Brussels sprouts will be lightly browned and wilted. Transfer the cooked Brussels sprouts to a large plate and squeeze the lemon wedges on top to serve.

491.Ritzy Pimento And Almond Turkey Casserole

Servings:4
Cooking Time: 32 Minutes
Ingredients:
- 1 pound (454 g) turkey breasts
- 1 tablespoon olive oil
- 2 boiled eggs, chopped
- 2 tablespoons chopped pimentos
- ¼ cup slivered almonds, chopped
- ¼ cup mayonnaise
- ½ cup diced celery
- 2 tablespoons chopped green onion
- ¼ cup cream of chicken soup
- ¼ cup bread crumbs

- Salt and ground black pepper, to taste

Directions:
1. Put the turkey breasts in a large bowl. Sprinkle with salt and ground black pepper and drizzle with olive oil. Toss to coat well.
2. Transfer the turkey to the air fryer basket.
3. Put the air fryer basket on the baking pan and slide into Rack Position 2, select Air Fry, set temperature to 390ºF (199ºC) and set time to 12 minutes.
4. Flip the turkey halfway through.
5. When cooking is complete, the turkey should be well browned.
6. Remove the turkey breasts from the oven and cut into cubes, then combine the chicken cubes with eggs, pimentos, almonds, mayo, celery, green onions, and chicken soup in a large bowl. Stir to mix.
7. Pour the mixture into the baking pan, then spread with bread crumbs.
8. Slide the baking pan into Rack Position 1, select Convection Bake, set time to 20 minutes.
9. When cooking is complete, the eggs should be set.
10. Remove from the oven and serve immediately.

492.Air Fried Blistered Tomatoes

Servings:4 To 6
Cooking Time: 10 Minutes
Ingredients:
- 2 pounds (907 g) cherry tomatoes
- 2 tablespoons olive oil
- 2 teaspoons balsamic vinegar
- ½ teaspoon salt
- ½ teaspoon ground black pepper

Directions:
1. Toss the cherry tomatoes with olive oil in a large bowl to coat well. Pour the tomatoes in the baking pan.
2. Put the air fryer basket on the baking pan and slide into Rack Position 2, select Air Fry, set temperature to 400ºF (205ºC) and set time to 10 minutes.
3. Stir the tomatoes halfway through the cooking time.
4. When cooking is complete, the tomatoes will be blistered and lightly wilted.
5. Transfer the blistered tomatoes to a large bowl and toss with balsamic vinegar, salt, and black pepper before serving.

493.Chocolate Buttermilk Cake

Servings:8
Cooking Time: 20 Minutes
Ingredients:
- 1 cup all-purpose flour
- ²/₃ cup granulated white sugar
- ¼ cup unsweetened cocoa powder

- ¾ teaspoon baking soda
- ¼ teaspoon salt
- ²/₃ cup buttermilk
- 2 tablespoons plus 2 teaspoons vegetable oil
- 1 teaspoon vanilla extract
- Cooking spray

Directions:
1. Spritz the baking pan with cooking spray.
2. Combine the flour, cocoa powder, baking soda, sugar, and salt in a large bowl. Stir to mix well.
3. Mix in the buttermilk, vanilla, and vegetable oil. Keep stirring until it forms a grainy and thick dough.
4. Scrape the chocolate batter from the bowl and transfer to the pan, level the batter in an even layer with a spatula.
5. Slide the baking pan into Rack Position 1, select Convection Bake, set temperature to 325ºF (163ºC) and set time to 20 minutes.
6. After 15 minutes, remove the pan from the oven. Check the doneness. Return the pan to the oven and continue cooking.
7. When done, a toothpick inserted in the center should come out clean.
8. Invert the cake on a cooling rack and allow to cool for 15 minutes before slicing to serve.

494.Enchilada Sauce

Servings: 2 Cups
Cooking Time: 0 Minutes
Ingredients:
- 3 large ancho chiles, stems and seeds removed, torn into pieces
- 1½ cups very hot water
- 2 garlic cloves, peeled and lightly smashed
- 2 tablespoons wine vinegar
- 1½ teaspoons sugar
- ½ teaspoon dried oregano
- ½ teaspoon ground cumin
- 2 teaspoons kosher salt or 1 teaspoon fine salt

Directions:
1. Mix together the chile pieces and hot water in a bowl and let stand for 10 to 15 minutes.
2. Pour the chiles and water into a blender jar. Fold in the garlic, vinegar, sugar, oregano, cumin, and salt and blend until smooth.
3. Use immediately.

495.Greek Frittata

Servings:2
Cooking Time: 8 Minutes
Ingredients:
- 1 cup chopped mushrooms
- 2 cups spinach, chopped
- 4 eggs, lightly beaten

- 3 ounces (85 g) feta cheese, crumbled
- 2 tablespoons heavy cream
- A handful of fresh parsley, chopped
- Salt and ground black pepper, to taste
- Cooking spray

Directions:
1. Spritz the baking pan with cooking spray.
2. Whisk together all the ingredients in a large bowl. Stir to mix well.
3. Pour the mixture in the prepared baking pan.
4. Slide the baking pan into Rack Position 1, select Convection Bake, set temperature to 350ºF (180ºC) and set time to 8 minutes.
5. Stir the mixture halfway through.
6. When cooking is complete, the eggs should be set.
7. Serve immediately.

496.Cauliflower And Pumpkin Casserole

Servings:6
Cooking Time: 50 Minutes
Ingredients:
- 1 cup chicken broth
- 2 cups cauliflower florets
- 1 cup canned pumpkin purée
- ¼ cup heavy cream
- 1 teaspoon vanilla extract
- 2 large eggs, beaten
- $^1/_3$ cup unsalted butter, melted, plus more for greasing the pan
- ¼ cup sugar
- 1 teaspoon fine sea salt
- Chopped fresh parsley leaves, for garnish
- TOPPING:
- ½ cup blanched almond flour
- 1 cup chopped pecans
- $^1/_3$ cup unsalted butter, melted
- ½ cup sugar

Directions:
1. Pour the chicken broth in the baking pan, then add the cauliflower.
2. Slide the baking pan into Rack Position 1, select Convection Bake, set temperature to 350ºF (180ºC) and set time to 20 minutes.
3. When cooking is complete, the cauliflower should be soft.
4. Meanwhile, combine the ingredients for the topping in a large bowl. Stir to mix well.
5. Pat the cauliflower dry with paper towels, then place in a food processor and pulse with pumpkin purée, heavy cream, vanilla extract, eggs, butter, sugar, and salt until smooth.
6. Clean the baking pan and grease with more butter, then pour the purée mixture in the pan. Spread the topping over the mixture.
7. Put the baking pan back to the oven. Select Bake and set time to 30 minutes.

8. When baking is complete, the topping of the casserole should be lightly browned.
9. Remove the casserole from the oven and serve with fresh parsley on top.

497.Fried Dill Pickles With Buttermilk Dressing

Servings:6 To 8
Cooking Time: 8 Minutes
Ingredients:
- Buttermilk Dressing:
- ¼ cup buttermilk
- ¼ cup chopped scallions
- ¾ cup mayonnaise
- ½ cup sour cream
- ½ teaspoon cayenne pepper
- ½ teaspoon onion powder
- ½ teaspoon garlic powder
- 1 tablespoon chopped chives
- 2 tablespoons chopped fresh dill
- Kosher salt and ground black pepper, to taste
- Fried Dill Pickles:
- ¾ cup all-purpose flour
- 1 (2-pound / 907-g) jar kosher dill pickles, cut into 4 spears, drained
- 2½ cups panko bread crumbs
- 2 eggs, beaten with 2 tablespoons water
- Kosher salt and ground black pepper, to taste
- Cooking spray

Directions:
1. Combine the ingredients for the dressing in a bowl. Stir to mix well.
2. Wrap the bowl in plastic and refrigerate for 30 minutes or until ready to serve.
3. Pour the flour in a bowl and sprinkle with salt and ground black pepper. Stir to mix well. Put the bread crumbs in a separate bowl. Pour the beaten eggs in a third bowl.
4. Dredge the pickle spears in the flour, then into the eggs, and then into the panko to coat well. Shake the excess off.
5. Arrange the pickle spears in a single layer in the air fryer basket and spritz with cooking spray.
6. Put the air fryer basket on the baking pan and slide into Rack Position 2, select Air Fry, set temperature to 400ºF (205ºC) and set time to 8 minutes.
7. Flip the pickle spears halfway through the cooking time.
8. When cooking is complete, remove from the oven.
9. Serve the pickle spears with buttermilk dressing.

498.Keto Cheese Quiche

Servings:8

Cooking Time: 1 Hour
Ingredients:
- Crust:
- 1¼ cups blanched almond flour
- 1 large egg, beaten
- 1¼ cups grated Parmesan cheese
- ¼ teaspoon fine sea salt
- Filling:
- 4 ounces (113 g) cream cheese
- 1 cup shredded Swiss cheese
- $1/_3$ cup minced leeks
- 4 large eggs, beaten
- ½ cup chicken broth
- ⅛ teaspoon cayenne pepper
- ¾ teaspoon fine sea salt
- 1 tablespoon unsalted butter, melted
- Chopped green onions, for garnish
- Cooking spray

Directions:
1. Spritz the baking pan with cooking spray.
2. Combine the flour, egg, Parmesan, and salt in a large bowl. Stir to mix until a satiny and firm dough forms.
3. Arrange the dough between two grease parchment papers, then roll the dough into a $1/_{16}$-inch thick circle.
4. Make the crust: Transfer the dough into the prepared pan and press to coat the bottom.
5. Slide the baking pan into Rack Position 1, select Convection Bake, set temperature to 325ºF (163ºC) and set time to 12 minutes.
6. When cooking is complete, the edges of the crust should be lightly browned.
7. Meanwhile, combine the ingredient for the filling, except for the green onions in a large bowl.
8. Pour the filling over the cooked crust and cover the edges of the crust with aluminum foil.
9. Slide the baking pan into Rack Position 1, select Convection Bake, set time to 15 minutes.
10. When cooking is complete, reduce the heat to 300ºF (150ºC) and set time to 30 minutes.
11. When cooking is complete, a toothpick inserted in the center should come out clean.
12. Remove from the oven and allow to cool for 10 minutes before serving.

499.Sweet And Sour Peanuts

Servings:9
Cooking Time: 5 Minutes

Ingredients:
- 3 cups shelled raw peanuts
- 1 tablespoon hot red pepper sauce
- 3 tablespoons granulated white sugar

Directions:
1. Put the peanuts in a large bowl, then drizzle with hot red pepper sauce and sprinkle with sugar. Toss to coat well.
2. Pour the peanuts in the air fryer basket.
3. Put the air fryer basket on the baking pan and slide into Rack Position 2, select Air Fry, set temperature to 400ºF (205ºC) and set time to 5 minutes.
4. Stir the peanuts halfway through the cooking time.
5. When cooking is complete, the peanuts will be crispy and browned. Remove from the oven and serve immediately.

500.Lush Seafood Casserole

Servings:2
Cooking Time: 22 Minutes

Ingredients:
- 1 tablespoon olive oil
- 1 small yellow onion, chopped
- 2 garlic cloves, minced
- 4 ounces (113 g) tilapia pieces
- 4 ounces (113 g) rockfish pieces
- ½ teaspoon dried basil
- Salt and ground white pepper, to taste
- 4 eggs, lightly beaten
- 1 tablespoon dry sherry
- 4 tablespoons cheese, shredded

Directions:
1. Heat the olive oil in a nonstick skillet over medium-high heat until shimmering.
2. Add the onion and garlic and sauté for 2 minutes or until fragrant.
3. Add the tilapia, rockfish, basil, salt, and white pepper to the skillet. Sauté to combine well and transfer them into the baking pan.
4. Combine the eggs, sherry and cheese in a large bowl. Stir to mix well. Pour the mixture in the baking pan over the fish mixture.
5. Slide the baking pan into Rack Position 1, select Convection Bake, set temperature to 360ºF (182ºC) and set time to 20 minutes.
6. When cooking is complete, the eggs should be set and the casserole edges should be lightly browned.
7. Serve immediately.

CPSIA information can be obtained
at www.ICGtesting.com
Printed in the USA
LVHW020727070121
675635LV00011B/488